THE
POWER
OF THE
HEALING
FIELD

"Brilliantly challenges our deepest-held beliefs about the nature of consciousness. Through rigorous documentation in case reports and practical, lucid explanations, Peter Mark Adams empowers us with a new set of tools and contexts to practically code and recode our reality, heal our ancestral past, understand the paranormal, and move through each moment with ethical intentionality."

ALEXANDER ETH, HOST OF THE *GLITCH BOTTLE* PODCAST

"As one in search of the lost consciousness technologies of the ancients, I thoroughly enjoyed this book. Peter reveals the multidimensionality of the human being by skillfully mapping the energy field of intelligence supported by groundbreaking scientists such as Rupert Sheldrake. His rational and logical methodology delivers a solid melding of scientific theories and energy healing that questions the terms of existence in which the scientific world operates. What makes this book a page-turner is the collection of real-life energy healing cases. Packed with mystery and wonderment, perhaps the most powerful thing about this book is that Peter provides hope by expanding what is possible on one's own healing journey."

VANESE MCNEILL, EXECUTIVE PRODUCER OF THE
MAGICAL EGYPT DOCUMENTARY SERIES

"*The Power of the Healing Field* outlines a new horizon of possibilities of controlling our awareness. The examples of the usage of psychic energy explained in the book illuminate the dark areas of our subconscious fears and help us to overcome the inherent fear of the infinite and impersonal. This is a very timely book that I would recommend to all thoughtful readers."

ALINA KIPREY, PROPRIETOR OF THE
ESOTERIC PUBLISHING HOUSE INVERTED TREE

"Peter Mark Adams provides a much-needed, inspiring exploration of energy healing and the ways its successes challenge the materialist assumptions of our culture. *The Power of the Healing Field* is a paradigm-shifting work, and I highly recommend it for everyone drawn to the healing arts and wider ways of knowing and interacting with spirit."

"Peter Mark Adams continues to impress with the breadth of experience he brings to the topic and his ability to present it clearly and concisely. This is a fine book for beginners as their foundation will be well established, and equally, experienced healers will find it insightful and practical. There is truly something for everyone in these pages."

"As a careful researcher and spellbinding nonfiction author, Peter Mark Adams's star has been on the rise and continuing to climb with each new offering. His unflinching willingness to tackle issues relating to the blind spots and limitations of modern Western thinking and some much-needed course corrections for modern Western science and technology are handled with his characteristic clarity, brilliance, and a frankness that is rare in this age. This book is an eyes-wide-open presentation of the very furthest frontiers of what modern science has discovered about the governing fields and invisible forces that organize the physical realm, the invisible causal movers, and primary influencers of biology. The insights offered in this book may hold the key to pulling humanity back from the brink of self-imposed annihilation, a much-needed cause to take pause and to reexamine the presumptions that have led us to this precarious state we find ourselves in."

THE
POWER
OF THE
HEALING FIELD

ENERGY MEDICINE, PSI ABILITIES,
AND ANCESTRAL HEALING

PETER MARK ADAMS

Healing Arts Press
Rochester, Vermont

Healing Arts Press
One Park Street
Rochester, Vermont 05767
www.HealingArtsPress.com

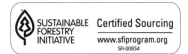

Text stock is SFI certified

Healing Arts Press is a division of Inner Traditions International

Originally published in 2014 by Balboa Press under the title *The Healing Field*

Note to the reader: *This book is intended as an informational guide. The remedies,
approaches, and techniques described herein are meant to supplement, and not to be a
substitute for, professional medical care or treatment. They should not be used to treat
a serious ailment without prior consultation with a qualified health care professional.*

Cataloging-in-Publication Data for this title is available from the Library of Congress

ISBN 978-1-64411-358-5 (print)
ISBN 978-1-64411-359-2 (ebook)

Printed and bound in the United States by Lake Book Manufacturing, Inc.
The text stock is SFI certified. The Sustainable Forestry Initiative® program
promotes sustainable forest management.

10 9 8 7 6 5 4 3 2 1

Text design and layout by Priscilla Harris Baker
This book was typeset in Garamond Premier Pro with Gill Sans, Minion, Bodoni
Ornaments, and Posterama used as display typefaces
Artwork by Peter Mark Adams

To send correspondence to the author of this book, mail a first-class letter to the
author c/o Inner Traditions • Bear & Company, One Park Street, Rochester, VT
05767, and we will forward the communication, or contact the author directly at
petermarkadams.com.

For Gülcan

Contents

Illustrations

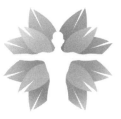

Acknowledgments

Very special thanks are owed to all those healers who freely shared their knowledge and case studies, and to all the people who offered accounts of their private experiences. Many thanks to Michael and Richard Greenwood for allowing me to use one of their illustrations. Last but not least, a very special thanks to my wife, life partner, and a great healer, Gülcan Arpacıoğlu-Adams, known as Kenzie, formerly an industrial engineer before dedicating herself to the path of healing—for providing many of the healing cases I have used in this book. Thanks also for all of her patience and support during the long process of researching and writing this book.

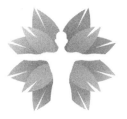

Introduction

The only courage that is demanded of us: to have courage for the most strange, the most singular, and the most inexplicable that we may encounter.

RAINER MARIA RILKE

THIS BOOK AROSE from a prolonged meditation on the diverse ways in which we experience healing and personal transformation. I have been lucky enough to undertake this journey in the company of my wife, Gülcan (Kenzie), and many other gifted healers and psychics who provided unstinting help and guidance. In the process I witnessed wonders that revealed a greatly expanded conception of self, reality, and our place within it. I found myself asking why it is that these things are so little known, so rarely experienced, and so obscured from view. Because many of these experiences possessed such rare and unusual qualities, I wanted to share them, since they suggest a far more expansive and uplifting view of who and what we are than what mainstream thinking allows for.

This book will help to illuminate these issues by dwelling on those aspects of reality that are the most controversial and the most challenging and difficult to find. Although this work is anchored in science, its subject matter occupies that twilight zone between objective science and subjective experience, between reason and intuition. All of the anomalous phenomena dealt with here are backed up by the records of our own case files and, as much as possible, by available scientific research. Above all I wanted to facilitate an understanding of the larger web of life and our place within it, for when we grasp this we begin to move toward a quality of understanding that relieves much of the fear, doubt, and uncertainty that overshadows the vast majority of people.

The Power of the Healing Field has been structured to progress from the day-to-day anomalies that many of us have experienced, toward the more unusual and, in some cases, disturbing phenomena that occur at the outermost edges of human experience. It is only by examining the full range of such experiences that we can grasp the hidden depths of reality and the true expanse of the human spirit.

In chapter 1, "Healing, Energy, and Consciousness," we set the scene by introducing the main categories and issues that we are going to deal with. In chapter 2, "Psi and Intuitive Knowledge," we look at how each and every one of us has the dynamic potential to access information with which we otherwise have no connection. In chapter 3, "Healing Issues within Our Timeline," we examine experiences from the extremities of our normal life cycle: those arising in the womb, during the birth process, and on the very brink of death. These experiences challenge the conventional understanding of consciousness and the boundaries of self-hood, of when the "I" can be said to exist. In chapter 4, "Healing Issues beyond Our Timeline," we extend our inquiry further, into the continuity of the self and the limits of consciousness, by examining examples of healing involving past lives as well as inherited family and ancestral trauma. Chapter 5, "The Healing Field," summarizes the implications of what we have learned up to now and proposes a model of consciousness and reality that allows us to make sense of these otherwise anomalous experiences. Chapter 6, "Healing on Extended Planes of Existence," expands our horizon yet again, to examine healing on levels of reality beyond the range of our immediate perceptual awareness. We consider the role of entity attachments of varying degrees of sentience that act to affect our health and mental balance. Chapter 7, "Healing through Spirit," considers mystical or peak experiences, including the variety of ways in which these are accessed and how they contribute to healing as well as the ethical and spiritual development of humanity. Finally, Chapter 8, "Conclusions," pulls all of this material together to develop an understanding of consciousness, reality, and identity that encompasses all of these phenomena. We then use this model to suggest strategies that will lead to profound levels of healing, increased happiness, and a greater contribution to our spiritual coevolution.

1

Healing, Energy, and Consciousness

When we heal ourselves, we heal the past, the present, and the future.

STEVEN D. FARMER

Almost two decades ago I was diagnosed by a medical doctor and acupuncturist with an enlarged liver. His diagnosis involved using a microhmmeter to monitor variations in the skin's electrical resistance on the main acupuncture meridian points. He told me that my condition could be healed, but this would require weekly treatments for the next eight months. A day or so later, Kenzie and I met a Russian bioenergist who offered to demonstrate her healing skills. Since neither of us shared a common language, we couldn't discuss my health issues or anything else for that matter. Instead, she passed her hands around me at a short distance from my body and quickly diagnosed the same liver condition as the acupuncturist had. This impressed both of us, and I decided to undertake a healing session with her the following week. The session started with her bringing her own energy into focus. She asked me to breathe deeply and rapidly a few times. I am familiar with various sorts of breathwork, so I recognized that this would quickly increase the level of my inner energy. She then massaged my liver, and this marked the last second at which my awareness could be said to be operating within normal bounds. She inhaled sharply. As she did so, her hands pulled some manner of blockage from my liver, as though she was ripping a plant, roots and all, out of the soil. I distinctly felt "it" move from me to her. She then exhaled powerfully over my head. Right then my whole mood and energy shifted. I felt weak and light at the same time.

Although these actions describe what happened, they completely fail to do justice to the intensity of the process that I experienced. When she pulled the problem out of me and into herself, it showed quite clearly in the pain and sadness that were etched on her face. A moment later, she lifted her face upward and powerfully blew out, permanently and completely releasing the problem. I felt weak. I lay down. All of a sudden I was completely overcome by what I can only describe as ecstatic bliss, pure and endless joy, a sense of the unutterable perfection and humor of existence itself. I dissolved in joyful laughter, a level and depth of laughter that I have never experienced before. I laughed uncontrollably for half an hour. About a week later, I visited the acupuncturist, who checked my liver once more only to find, much to his amazement, that he could no longer find any trace of the previous liver problem. When we told him about my session with the bioenergist, he said, "I must meet this woman!" Decades later I am still completely free of the problem.

This account touches on many of the themes that we will be exploring through the firsthand accounts of gifted energy healers. In particular, it illustrates the intimate connection that exists between our natural energy field, our health, and the quality of our awareness. It demonstrates our innate ability to intuitively understand the deep, emotional roots of ill health. And it shows us how natural processes can effect fast and effective healing by changing the dynamics of our energy field.

The Parameters of Reality and Consciousness

The reality revealed through energy-based healing is quite different from the world of most people's day-to-day experience. Like most of us, I have been raised to believe that what you see is all there is, and everything in the universe can be reduced to and explained by particles of matter bumping into one another. But the accounts of healing gathered here, drawn for the most part from our own case files, reveal that this picture is grossly inadequate. Reality is far more complex, multidimensional, and connected than we imagine. Each and every one of us, using only natural methods, can realize a level of healing and positive personal transformation far beyond conventional expectations.

Like almost everyone, I possess an inbuilt skepticism to any suggestion that reality is fundamentally different from what my day-to-day experience and mainstream science tells me. When challenged by anomalies that exceed this one-size-fits-all worldview, the response is usually one of ridicule, outright dismissal, or rationalization. However, there are very good reasons why a change in our worldview is long overdue. People are increasingly aware and accepting of the fact that their experience does not accord with mainstream science. Recently, one of the world's leading philosophers, Thomas Nagel, triggered a storm of criticism by stating the obvious fact that the five-hundred-year-old scientific project of attempting to explain everything in terms of interactions among the smallest particles, called *reductive materialism,* has failed.[1] A similar argument has been advanced by biologist and complexity theorist Stuart Kauffman.[2] It failed because it cannot account for the most defining and essential features of life: consciousness, agency, meaning, and values.

By *consciousness* we mean the irreducible, luminous awareness of the present moment shared by all sentient beings. It is sometimes hard to grasp, but this dynamic quality that so essentially defines us escapes all explanation, whether on the part of philosophy, neuroscience, psychology, or evolutionary theory. By *agency* we refer to the fundamental quality of intentionality that all sentient beings possess: our desiring, willing, planning, and executing. Purposeful action gives rise to meaning, another fundamental quality of being. And with meaningful action comes values. Values capture our inherent sensitivity toward such fundamental issues as right and wrong, justice and injustice. We all know that these essential elements are characteristic of all sentient life and form an intrinsic part of reality, and yet modern science can find no place for them.

Where we do find these qualities at their most pronounced is in the arena of healing and personal and spiritual transformation. For this reason we need to remain open to the possibility that anomalous experiences in these contexts, such as those that accompanied my own healing, may well be pointing us toward a broader conception of reality and consciousness than has been accepted up till now.

Indeed, many of the cases described in this book, involving intense grief and trauma, were chosen from among the many thousands of cases in our files precisely because they challenge our notions of reality, consciousness, and the possible when it comes to healing a broad range of physical, mental, and emotional problems.

What may well come as a surprise to those who have hitherto not been exposed to energy healing is the rapidity with which even the most extreme effects can be resolved once their originating nexus has been identified. We can better understand how these remarkable cases are possible if we understand the process involved a little better. The great skill of the energy healer lies in three closely related aptitudes: first, the ability to facilitate the person's own identification of the precise causal nexus of their disturbance; second, assisting the person in retaining a focus on their feelings without reliving them in all their intensity; and third, applying the energy healing protocol persistently, either by the healer, or by facilitating the person's own use of it, until the negative emotions and any others that emerge in connection with the original trauma are wholly eliminated. This third component, the actual application of the energy healing protocol, is by far the simplest and easiest part of the healing process to learn and apply, and its results are experienced almost immediately as positively beneficial. Most of the various energy healing protocols available today can deliver relief from a range of mental, emotional, and physical problems. When facilitated by an experienced healer they can achieve a success rate upward of 90 percent. In our practice over the years we have had medical doctors, psychiatrists, psychotherapists, and professional coaches undergo training with us so that they can add energy healing to their professional practice as an adjunct therapeutic technique.

The process by which we come to hold our beliefs about the nature of reality, consciousness, and personal identity—our enculturation or programming—prepares us to fit in with a certain society and culture. But just because it enables us to interact with the portion of reality relevant to our society does not mean that it also prepares us for perceiving those aspects of reality beyond our society's sphere of interest. For this we require a much broader perspective: the capacity to push the boundaries of consensual understanding and accommodate a fresh vision of the familiar world we inhabit. I liken this process to deprogramming.

My own deprogramming has been a continuing process over many years. One event that helped me occurred when I was growing up in Africa in the early 1960s. We had decided to drive down to the coast, some four hundred miles away. Pedro, who worked with my father, hitched a ride with us. We drove down from the Kenyan highlands through the great Rift Valley and then headed southeast. All day we traveled on the rough red earth road that in those years ran all the way to the coast. We crossed dried-up riverbeds and vast tracks of featureless savannah, a great plume of red dust flowing out behind the car. Late that day we arrived on the edge of the city of Mombasa on the coast. We stopped at a small open market next to the road to pick up some fruit before going on to our final destination much further to the south. As we got out of the car, a younger, casually dressed man who was beaming from ear to ear stepped forward and warmly greeted Pedro. It was his brother!

We asked Pedro how on earth his brother could possibly be waiting for him at such a remote place on that day and time. He shrugged. "Because I would be here," he said, as though it was the most normal thing to expect! In the early 1960s, the internet and mobile phones were still twenty-five years or so in the future. And even supposing Pedro had phoned him sometime before we set off, it still doesn't explain his brother being at that particular roadside market at that very time, and our spontaneous decision to stop there. Is there more to reality than we can possibly imagine? As we explore the various cases presented here, we will see that the answer is a resounding yes!

Another event that helped me to remain open to new possibilities occurred in my teens. I had joined a karate club run by a highly respected master, Ronnie Colwell. One night Ronnie demonstrated the controlled use of chi, or vital energy. He had a few of the burlier club members hold three thick wooden boards, each around 12 inches (30 cm) square and around 2.5 inches (6.4 cm) thick, tightly together. He then struck the first board. Nothing happened. But when we examined the boards we found that while the first and second boards showed no sign of damage, the third board, the one farthest away from the strike, was neatly split down the middle. How he did this, how it was even possible, puzzled most of us at the time. It still does today, over forty years later. The martial artist's explanation is that it is done by focusing their chi on a point beyond where they are going to strike. In this case, Ronnie focused his energy on the third board, the one farthest away from the struck surface, and then split it.

Finally, perhaps the most dramatic experience that confirmed my acceptance of an esoteric worldview occurred on the cusp of my entry to the world of energy healing. When Kenzie and I met our first Reiki teacher we sat and talked about energy and the path to inner cleansing and personal cultivation. After a while I started to feel that there was something wrong with my eyes. I became aware of stray blues and greens that appeared to flow across portions of our teacher's hands and arms. I rubbed my eyes and checked what I was seeing outside the window.

No trace of the stray colors appeared—it seemed that my eyes were not at fault. I resumed concentrating on what she was saying, only for the colors to spread and grow more vibrant. I tried a number of times to shake off the visual "distortion", but by now the phenomenon had taken on a life of its own—the colors had formed a kaleidoscope! The disconnected patches of color began to coalesce into a seamless field of green streaked with deep blue that flowed across her hands, arms, and—finally—her entire body, swirling in graceful eddies like oil paint over the surface of water. I became aware that these colors radiated ten to fifteen centimeters out from her body, forming an iridescent field of emerald. I described what I was seeing to Kenzie, and this confirmed that we were on the right track to study with this teacher. When I reflect on my experience, over twenty years later, it occurs to me that I was able to see her aura so easily because she had a very high level of inner energy. The controlled activation and ascent of this inner energy is one of the main aims of most yogic systems. Apparently, our talk about aspiration for healing and growth raised my level of awareness and this enabled me to see her aura.

The reality of chi and of our wider energy fields is apparent to those who practice the martial arts, the many forms of spiritual yoga, or any of the energy-based healing modalities. We will return to consider the nature of these energies and the evidence for them later. For now let's agree to call the energy surrounding all sentient beings *biofield energy,* to distinguish it from the conventional forms of electromagnetic energy produced by every organ and part of our bodies.

As we saw in my own case of healing, a gifted healer can intuitively access a deeper, more perceptive understanding of health problems than would be apparent to most of us. Such extraperceptual skills are regarded as psychic abilities. This is just one manifestation of a range of abilities subsumed under the concept of *psi.* Because of the centrality of these abilities to many types of healing processes, we will examine them in greater detail in the next chapter. The insights that arise because of a healer's innate psychism, or psi abilities, involve shifting awareness beyond the normal range of the waking state. Such shifts are commonly called *altered states of consciousness.*

Altered States of Consciousness

In every society and in every age, people have engaged in practices that shift their awareness to take in a much broader spectrum of reality. In the West we call these shifts *altered states,* and until fairly recently we have tended to dismiss them as psychological distortions or even as pathologies. But in many societies, and among those dedicated to a broad range of healing and spiritual development practices, these shifts, and the realities they provide access to, form a vital part of everyday life. Our ability to sense things hidden from normal perception is far more dynamic than many of us imagine.

In the 1960s the term *altered states of consciousness* was increasingly used by psychologists such as Arnold Ludwig and Charles T. Tart, and anthropologists like Stanley Krippner, to categorize the much broader range of experiences arising from their research, especially in non-Western societies. *Altered states* were initially defined as any state that exhibited "sufficient deviation"[3] or a "qualitative shift"[4] or "difference" from "normal waking consciousness."[5] But definitions like these beg the question: What constitutes "sufficient," and who is to judge what is "normal"? Not only definitions like these but also the very need for such a category have been challenged by people from cultures who still use a much fuller spectrum of awareness. Jane Middleton-Moz, an Indigenous American author and academic, challenged psychiatrist Stanislav Grof, one of the founders and the chief theoretician of transpersonal psychology, on precisely this point: "I don't understand why you use the term *nonordinary states.* For my people, these experiences are part of the normal spectrum of human experience!"[6]

In some ways the idea of altered states tells us more about the limitations of our own culture than it does about the states themselves. States

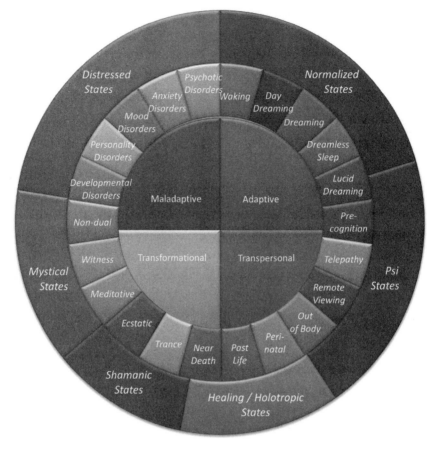

Figure 1.1. The spectrum of consciousness

of consciousness such as the various levels of wakefulness and sleep or certain meditative states are relatively discrete. They can be identified by their signature patterns of brain waves (alpha, beta, etc.) and the activation of specific areas of the brain. But we cannot say the same for altered states, which do not identify with any specific subjective experience or brain state. What, then, does an altered state signify? It can, of course, cover anything from psychosis to drunkenness, but in general usage an altered state refers to an extension or expansion of awareness that fulfills some specific purpose. In other words, the significance of altered states lies not in the neuroscience, psychology, or anthropology surrounding them, but in what they can do for us. In short, altered states provide alternative ways of engaging with reality. In all times and cultures, altered states have been used to provide access to information and realities not accessible by other means, to facilitate healing, survival, and as an integral part of spiritual transformation.

There are four basic contexts in which we see such shifts occurring: accessing remote information, healing, shamanism, and mysticism. None of these areas exclude the others, and they all exhibit a large degree of overlap. I have further characterized states of awareness that access remote information as *transpersonal.* This means that they are used to pick up information about distant, hidden, or lost objects, people, or events. I have characterized most of the healing, shamanic, and mystical states as *transformational,* since they often accompany, or even induce, profound healing and personal and spiritual change.

As we noted, many skilled healers intuitively access unconscious, forgotten, or hidden information that provides the key to their client's healing. These healers combine their access to such information with other skills that facilitate the integration of emotional upsets and traumas. Some of the more exotic examples include fetal, birth-related, ancestral, and past-life traumas. Practicing shamans combine psi and healing skills with additional abilities in working with a range of etheric, astral, nonhuman, and other-dimensional entities. Finally, mystics may combine all of these abilities with their connection to higher-order beings in order to realize and sustain transcendental levels of awareness.

To provide some context, we will use these categories to relate altered states to the more usual range of experiences, such as the various levels of wakefulness and sleep, and a few of the various classifications of mental disorders. The idea is not to create an exhaustive classification of every possible state of consciousness—an impossible undertaking—but rather to provide a model that helps us orient ourselves to this complex material. Finally, in the coming chapters, we will add some of the experiences typically associated with each of these states.

2

Psi and Intuitive Knowledge

A person experiences life as something separated from the rest—a kind of optical delusion of consciousness. Our task must be to free ourselves from this self-imposed prison, and through compassion, to find the reality of Oneness.

ALBERT EINSTEIN

Kenzie woke up one morning and said, "I can't stop thinking of Nursel. She's a friend of mine who moved to Canada. I haven't heard from her for nearly seven years. Her name is continuously on my mind." At odd times throughout the day she repeated this and remarked that she was waiting for some development related to her friend. Sure enough, that afternoon she called Kenzie. She was in town and wished to meet up.

ALTHOUGH SUCH EXPERIENCES form a normal part of everyday life, especially in the context of close relationships, conventional thinking is unwilling to reflect on the implications of such experiences in terms of our understanding of consciousness and reality. In fact, we are positively encouraged to dismiss them as mere coincidences, but anything that regularly works to produce actionable knowledge cannot be dismissed so easily.

Accessing Knowledge beyond the Five Senses

We all possess an innate capacity for psi, the ability to access information or influence events beyond the reach of our five senses. Such information may relate to the unknown past, to lost or hidden objects, and (though with many complications) the probability of specific future events. Most of us experience this ability as a sudden insight that breaks into the day-to-day flow of our thoughts. It often occurs when we least expect it, especially when we are in a relaxed, defocalized state of awareness. In such states we are far more open to registering emergent ideas and feelings. However, this kind of intuitive perception can also be deliberately induced. This is usually achieved through a combination of focusing on a specific piece of information and combining this with an otherwise relaxed and receptive state of mind.

The general term *clairvoyance* (literally, "clear vision") covers the various types of direct, unmediated perception concerning objects, people, or events that are beyond the reach of our own senses. The more usual types of psi phenomena include:

- **Premonition:** emotional awareness of some unspecified thing that is about to happen
- **Precognition:** knowledge of a specific event, often of a personally significant nature, that is about to occur
- **Retrocognition:** knowledge of an event that occurred in the past concerning which we lack any information
- **Telesthenia:** knowledge of objects, people, or events with which the observer has no connection whatsoever; more usually subsumed under the term *remote viewing*
- **Telepathy:** picking up information from another person or sentient being without sensory communication

The implications for the veracity of any of these forms of "knowing" for our understanding of consciousness and the nature of reality are, of course, enormous. However, the conditions under which these states of awareness tend to arise are so spontaneous and specific to particular people, times, and places as to make scientific replication and validation almost impossible. They represent a direct approach to the acquisition of knowledge that is more characteristic of and accepted by traditional, indigenous, and pre-modern societies and cultures. It is hardly surprising, therefore, that they are not accepted as valid by mainstream science. That said, just how widespread are reports of these phenomena?

Most people have experienced at least one of these forms of direct knowing at some point in their lives. A study of the phenomena by the American Society for Psychical Research (ASPR) found that over half of the population of the United States and Europe claim to have experienced telepathy, clairvoyance, or contact with the dead, though only a small percentage of people—around 10 percent—claim to have experienced all three. Overall, more women than men report having these experiences. Other factors, such as educational level, were found to be irrelevant.[1] A further survey found that two-thirds of the U.S. population claim to have had a psi or mystical experience. Intriguingly, as epidemiologist and senior research fellow for the National Institute for Healthcare Research (NIHR) Jeff Levin found, the incidence of these experiences is increasing with each successive generation.[2]

The frequency with which people experience such insights varies enormously. Some people make a living from their psi-related skills; others may have these experiences on an almost daily basis, and still others hardly ever, if at all. There appear to be many different factors at work. As with most activities, innate talent is important, but our openness to such possibilities and how we choose to develop our awareness is also crucial. If our attention is constantly absorbed by focused, analytical activity, we will tend to lack the receptivity needed to pick up on these more subtle indications.

Premonition and Precognition

One evening Kenzie and I went out to eat. After leaving the restaurant, we crossed the road to do some window-shopping (shoes and bags, as I recall). As I was waiting for her I was suddenly overcome by a sense of foreboding. I looked around the street and back across at the restaurant, but nothing was happening. I was puzzled. A minute later, a figure slipped out of an alley next to the restaurant and threw something onto its open terrace. There was a loud bang followed by the sound of breaking glass and people screaming. Luckily, no one was hurt, though many people were in a state of shock. We immediately went over to help out. We then understood that it had only been a sound bomb and not something far worse.

Premonitions such as this are an emotional response to or awareness of a future event—in this case, a potential threat for which there were no indications in our immediate sensory environment. Precognition, on the other hand, entails the much stronger claim to have actual knowledge of future events when there is otherwise no sensory proof. Now common sense tells us that since future events have not yet transpired, we cannot possibly have awareness of them. But before we deal with this objection, let's look at some of the available evidence and then return to consider the implications of it for our understanding of reality.

A range of experiments relating to premonition have been undertaken by biologist Rupert Sheldrake. One famous experiment involved pets who seem to know when their owners are returning home. Even with trips of up to fifteen kilometers from home, and with a randomly selected return time, pets seem to know both when their owner decides to return and when their return journey actually starts. The percentage of their time waiting at a window in anticipation of their owner's return increases proportionately. It jumps from around 15 percent of their time normally, to 25 percent during the ten minutes or so when the decision to return is being made, and up to 55 percent of their time once the journey home actually starts.[3]

As already noted, precognition involves a stronger claim: to actually know about a future event that could not otherwise be anticipated. A typical example is suddenly thinking of a certain person, only to have them call you or meet you a short time later. Another common example involves knowing who is calling you before you see the caller I.D. A Monash University survey found that 80 percent of people claimed to have experienced one or another of these forms of precognition.[4] They especially occur between people who share a deep emotional bond. Try asking twins or close siblings about their awareness of the other's emotional states, even when they are far apart. So common are such experiences that few of us stop to consider their radical implications for understanding the nature and interplay of consciousness and reality. Anything this widespread that exhibits such a high frequency and predictive accuracy can hardly be labeled a coincidence!

If we take these events at face value, as genuine examples of direct, intuitive knowledge, they represent a major challenge to the conventional understanding of consciousness and reality. The following story is fairly typical of Kenzie's intuitive approach using energy psychology techniques. These techniques, which are now used by coaches, healing professionals, doctors, psychotherapists, and psychiatrists worldwide, are mind-body approaches that combine behavioral therapy with somatic biofield therapy.

I was working with a client whose husband had died after a long and happy marriage. She had been unable to come to terms with his death and was overwhelmed with grief. As we sat together, a mental image came to me. It was of a man washing the dishes and cleaning up around the kitchen. There was a strong feeling of sadness and the message, "I don't want you to do this." I asked my client what significance, if any, this image and message had for her. She immediately answered that throughout their long marriage her husband had always insisted on doing the dishes, never allowing her do them. Since his death she had kept herself continuously busy in the kitchen, washing everything in sight, trying to connect with him. She understood that she had to give this up, and that he would be happier if she got on with her life. The image and the message helped her to clear her grief after using energy psychology techniques.

What was so significant in this session was that a piece of obscure, highly personal, but extremely precise information—the single piece of information necessary to trigger the healing process—occurred spontaneously to the healer at just the right time. Among experienced healers this happens quite frequently and is an integral part of their expertise. Hidden in such apparently small, mundane details are truths that should cause us to question our entire understanding of mind and our connections with the wider reality.

Dowsing and Remote Viewing

Up till now we have dealt with spontaneous access to information with which we have an emotional but not a physical connection. We will now turn to deliberate attempts to access information with which we have no connection whatsoever.

My first exposure to dowsing came one day when I returned to a summer house we had rented, to find a man purposefully wandering around the garden. He had a small, Y-shaped stick in his hands. He walked around the front of the house, turned, and then walked back around the side. He stopped and indicated a spot to the caretaker. I guessed they were busy with site management and left them to it. A week later, upon returning home, I was confronted by a flatbed truck reversed up the driveway; it had a crane mounted behind the cab and a mound of tubes on the back. At the side the house stood a twenty-meter derrick. Tubes ran down and into the ground at the spot the man had indicated the week before. From the hole in the ground, a great tide of mud oozed out and ran down the driveway and across the lawn. The man I had seen the week before had been a professional dowser. He had indicated a spot for drilling that would provide access to fresh water in what was otherwise a dry, barren landscape. The previous week he had announced that a good supply of fresh water would be found at a depth of 90 meters or so. The drilling crew hit fresh water at 110 meters.

Dowsing has traditionally been used to detect lost or hidden objects such as sources of water, oil, or minerals. Detection is often performed using a pendulum or dowsing rods. Such tools are not essential but they help the dowser to externalize the answer to any question they have asked. The dowsing response is intuitive, psychophysical feedback that arises in answer to a specific question. Concerning his own approach, Hamish Miller, a professional dowser, wrote, "It is all about tuning your mind. The aim is complete relaxation in body and thoughts, but keeping one tiny part of your mind totally concentrated on the target."[5]

The dowsing response is probably one of the most familiar and hence more acceptable forms of remote sensing practice. It is one that just about anyone can learn and develop. There is, however, a big gap between the performance levels of interested amateurs and the professionals who earn their living from their abilities. Is there any independent scientific evidence establishing the validity of this practice?

To assess the effectiveness of its foreign-aid contributions, the German government undertook a ten-year, multination study of the relative success rates of experienced dowsers in finding water as compared to conventional techniques. They found that the success rates of experienced dowsers were as high as 96 percent against an expected 30 to 50 percent using conventional techniques.[6] In addition, the dowsers were able to predict the depth and yield of a well to within 10 to 20 percent accuracy. This study was undertaken in areas of the world such as sub-Saharan Africa, where water sources are especially deep, and a deviation of just one meter either side could mean the difference between success and failure.

Dowsing is sometimes explained as an interaction between the dowsing rods and subtle variations in the earth's electromagnetic field resulting from subsurface features such as water or minerals. In this case the dowsing instrument is thought to act like an antenna that picks up and amplifies these subtle signals. There are two problems with this explanation, however. First, it is possible to dowse an area without a dowsing instrument of any kind; the "information" derived by the dowser can be intuited directly by paying attention to a specific "target," such as a water source and landscape or map, rather than "mediated through" a physiologically induced signal from a physical instrument. Second, it is possible to dowse an area remotely. This can be done, for example, by dowsing a map. In this case the possible contribution of the area's electromagnetic fields hardly arises.

An acquaintance of ours, Ali Seydi Gultekin, a geological engineer as well as a professional dowser, is often called on to provide a preliminary analysis of the water potential of plots of land situated on a different continent. He does this by dowsing with a pendulum the large aerial photographs of the plots that are sent to him. After selecting the most likely plots, he flies in to carry out a more detailed study on the ground. Some of the people using his services are interested in investing in hotels in the desert around Las Vegas, Nevada. They need to carefully evaluate the viability of underground water sources as a key element in managing the risk to the hundreds of millions dollars involved in such ventures. Their siting over ample, accessible sources of water is essential to their long-term viability. In his spare time he flies to Africa to work on a charitable basis locating and tapping supplies of underground water for remote villages.

Psi and the Limits of Knowledge

Most of us have experienced psi—psychic phenomena or powers—at one time or another, even if it is just thinking of someone, only to have them unexpectedly appear or call us. But at the core of the professional's expertise lies the ability to combine highly receptive modes of awareness with a focused intent to locate some specific object. Their focused intent is sufficient to filter out everything that doesn't fit their search criteria. In other words, the psi faculty operates as an open, intentionally directed search and locate mechanism with nonlocal capabilities. By *nonlocal* I mean an object or event with which we have no physical connection. This may be because it is lost in the past, relates to the future, is hidden, unconscious, or undisclosed. But if we have no physical connection with the source of the information, given the cases that we have looked at, we must have some other connection with it. Understanding the nature of this connection takes us to the very heart of the issue of what consciousness is. I suggest that psi is a defining property of consciousness.

Neuroanthropologist Charles Laughlin has noted that many societies accept as verifiable knowledge the information derived from different states of consciousness. This includes psi, intuition, dreams, and visions. He calls these cultures "polyphasic" and contrasts them with those societies whose culture is largely "monophasic," that is, cultures that only credit as knowledge the information that is derived in normal waking consciousness.[7] But as we saw, even in the most monophasic of secular societies, a large and growing segment of the population is willing to accept as knowledge the kind of information derived from states of intuitive and empathic awareness. Outside of academia, mainstream science, and the media, the grassroots of Western culture remains in many ways profoundly polyphasic. The majority of people honor a variety of ways in which things can come to be known, though they tend to draw the line at information derived from the more extreme end of the spectrum, such as prophecy and divination.

Why Is Psi So Important?

Philosopher Charles Taylor identifies the characteristic sense of disengagement from and disenchantment with many aspects of life—which is at the heart of so many of our modern ills—as rooted in a loss of "porosity" in relation to our selfhood. This refers to the openness, relatedness, and "enchantment" that comes through engaging empathically with life on its many different levels.[8]

The ability to feel connected to all life-forms is the key to our continued personal and spiritual development. It is also the key to our continued survival as a species. Humanity is challenged to move beyond the unconscious demonization of other groups, peoples, and cultures and its indifference to the destruction and pollution of the natural environment. Around the world, the forces of globalization and industrialization are eroding both biological and cultural diversity. We encounter the same brands, clothing, entertainment, and food products wherever we go. Less commented on is the fact that this uniform consumer culture, which represents a loss of cultural diversity, tends to undermine perceptual diversity, which is our natural ability to connect to reality using different states of awareness. By relating to others in an intuitive and empathic way, perceptual diversity implies a far more holistic engagement with reality. As environmental and medical anthropologist Tara Lumpkin has pointed out, it is easy to see how such states play an important role in retaining harmony and balance in our own lives, in society, and in the environment.[9] She points out that all three losses of diversity (biological, cultural, and perceptual) are closely related. Once we open the door, so to speak, to other ways of knowing, when we accept that these states provide access to a broader, more connected understanding of reality, then our entire conception of the relationship between self and the environment has to change.[10]

Holistic, intuitive, and empathic ways of relating to reality are often thought of as sacrificing objectivity in favor of imagination or guesswork. In other words, information gained in these ways, even if it turns out to be true, can't qualify as knowledge. The classical definition of knowledge, one that has been around for at least twenty-five hundred years, defines knowledge as justified true belief. This formula has been passed down, unchanged, from Plato[11] to modern-day philosophy.[12] But because of the way in which our concept of justification has evolved over the last five hundred years or so, both intuitive and direct knowledge are thought of as lacking justification, that is, lacking causal linkages that can be independently demonstrated and reproduced by others. Intuitive and direct knowledge fail to meet these criteria for the simple reason that they depend on each person's ability to access these special forms of perception. But as we saw in the German government study, the success rates of professional dowsers are consistently higher than those of conventional hydrologists. If these "softer" forms of knowing produce results that are right more often than they are wrong, and a whole lot better than those available through conventional means, then we need to revisit our understanding of what constitutes knowledge. Knowledge, relevant facts, and truth are as much determined by our cultural frame of reference as they are by what is "out there." The argument over the validity of psi is as much about how we, as a culture, frame our understanding as it is a debate about the evidence.

Developing our awareness in order to reliably access a much broader spectrum of reality has always required some degree of personal transformation. We find evidence of this among most of the world's remaining aboriginal peoples. Later we will examine one example, the Kalahari Kung healing dance.[13] This is a case that throws considerable light on evidence uncovered by archaeologist David Lewis-Williams for the use of altered states as early as 40,000 BCE, as seen in cave paintings and rock art.[14] Throughout the ancient Indo-Chinese, Asiatic, and Greco-Roman worlds, philosophy was closely tied to spiritual issues and involved a whole range of practical disciplines—from diet to contemplation—designed to effect personal transformation.[15] Based on his historical survey of the disciplines employed to effect personal and spiritual development in antiquity, philosopher Michel Foucault concluded that "the philosophical theme 'how to have access to the truth' and the question of spirituality (what transformations in the being of the subject are necessary for access to the truth) were never separate."[16]

These ancient conceptions survived in Europe, though in an increasingly marginalized form, until at least the seventeenth century, when the emergence of a worldview predicated wholly on the scientific method supplanted them. The benefit of this shift was that it cleared the way for the rapid advances in science and technology that we see continuing today. However, it also resulted in an enormous flattening of our perspective on and insight into ourselves, as well as a profound loss of connectedness with certain subtle, less obvious aspects of reality. One of the purposes of this book is to help heal this breach and reestablish the older model of direct knowing alongside our modern conception.

A New Model of Consciousness and Reality

From this brief overview of some of the experiential and scientific evidence of psi we can draw a number of conclusions. First and foremost, we need to remember that the challenge psi presents is not a challenge to science. It is, however, a challenge to the mainstream scientific understanding of consciousness and reality. The most extreme of these cases involves emotional reactions to or knowledge of future events. How can we sense or have knowledge of events that have yet to occur? In what possible sense could such events be said to exist? And yet, as we have seen, numerous scientific experiments and many firsthand experiences confirm that this is exactly what happens. If we accept the validity of these experiences, then surely we must find ourselves in conflict with both common sense and scientific conceptions of time.

The disparity between our day-to-day experiences and our experience of consciousness and reality as revealed by our engagement with psi is so great that it should give us pause for thought. Is there something missing in mainstream understanding? Our present moment of awareness is always a momentary snapshot, the self's unique point of view. But if, as the evidence suggests, our awareness can be spatially and temporally displaced or refocused to access different times and places or to intercept another's thoughts, feelings, and memories, then we surely need a different model of consciousness and its relationship to reality. Perhaps by examining the most extreme, rare, and subtle manifestations of awareness we can begin to discern the outlines of what this model might look like.

From an experiential point of view we can think of intuitive perception as arising from a movement or shift in our awareness within a broader spectrum of consciousness whose composition and boundaries we have yet to fully understand. This movement is experienced as a progressive broadening of our awareness and a corresponding shrinking of our sense of a discrete, biographically constructed self. The progressive broadening of our awareness moves through a spectrum of defocalized states. We can categorize these states in a number of ways, such as the following sequence, which represents just one way of doing so. This sequence runs from present-moment awareness through instinctive, intuitive, empathic, and psychic modes. This scale is experienced by most of us, though states above the level of empathic become progressively rarer.

With the broadening of our awareness, the solidity of our orientation to the here and now, our connectedness to mundane reality, and

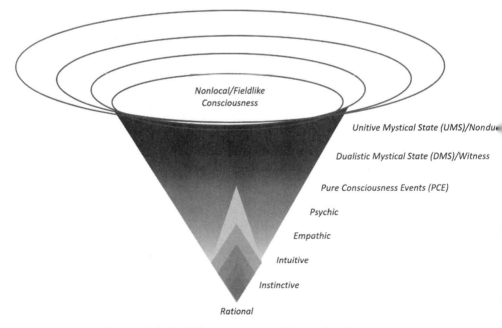

Figure 2.1. Fieldlike structure of defocalized awareness

our sense of selfhood begins to dissolve. With this dissolution we can access nonlocal information, that is, information from beyond the boundaries of our immediate senses. As we have seen, this information may relate to events, people, or objects with which we have no physical connection. Beyond these modes, certain psychic modes of awareness become accessible. Among very gifted healers, many of whom can access this level of awareness, information about the energy body, the deep emotional causes of ill health and misfortune, and the effects of past lives become transparent. Progressing beyond these psychic modes of awareness we begin to access the states of unitive and nondual awareness characteristic of the world's mystical traditions. Our awareness may come to feel oceanic. And like any fathomless space it arouses both our curiosity and our fear, for the limitless, like the formless, threatens to entirely engulf our sense of identity.

The ability to experience these states is a natural one, albeit one that is innately stronger in some people. It is therefore an ability that can be developed through training. We have seen that under suitable conditions it provides a path to direct knowledge and understanding. In the next chapter we will see how these states of knowing can access deep memory (that is, remembrances that run back through our biographical timeline to include past lives and ancestral memories that directly affect our health and well-being).

3

Healing Issues within Our Timeline

Be watchful—the grace of God appears suddenly. It comes without warning to an open heart.

RUMI

IN THIS CHAPTER we will deal with healing issues within the biographical timeline, that is, between conception and death. By looking at some of the more unusual cases that we have on file we will start to explore the limits and nature of consciousness and the boundaries of personal identity.

John was a successful aspiring manager with a large multinational corporation. His natural grace, good manners, and generosity marked him as someone most people would like to know. But appearances can belie the suffering that overshadows many people's inner lives. John came to me suffering from deep-seated, persistent feelings of loneliness, feelings that haunted him no matter where he was or whose company he was in. He wanted to see whether rebirthing breathwork would help him.

Rebirthing Breathwork is a personal development modality that uses circular breathing, *in which the inhale is connected with the exhale, to heighten one's inner energy, gain access to a greatly expanded level of awareness, and facilitate the integration of emotional issues.*

The sessions are conducted lying down to support the fullest level of relaxation. During his third session John suddenly started moving violently. From a lying position he jerked up and down from the waist and from side to side, as though trying to escape from some tight confinement. Finally his movements subsided. He experienced cold, darkness, and feelings of abandonment and loneliness. Suddenly he sat up and announced, "It's done!" He felt clear and focused. Something had clearly integrated at a very deep level. I later learned that when still in his mother's womb, his mother's waters had broken and she had been unable to get to a hospital for many hours. Unable to commence the birth process, the baby experienced the womb as a dark, cold, lonely place. It was this experience that had haunted him throughout his life and that had now resurfaced, to be integrated during the rebirthing session. The powerful movements back and forth reenacted those of the baby trying to get free of the womb before exhaustion and a sense of overwhelming loneliness overcame him. In the following weeks, John searched carefully for any traces of his former deep-seated loneliness, but of the feelings that had haunted him all of his life, not a trace remained.

When Do "We" Begin?

We normally think of the source of emotional disturbances as occurring in childhood. But some troubles appear to have much deeper roots. As we see in John's case, significant life issues can be connected to the nature of our birth process. Problems at this stage routinely surface, and are resolved, during Rebirthing Breathwork. But as we will see, some issues have their origins far earlier. The following cases are drawn from Kenzie's files.

Anne was a well-educated professional in her forties who was troubled by her continuing codependency with her mother. Despite the fact that she had lived abroad independently for many years, educating herself and establishing a career, she still felt compelled to return to her home country in order to be closer to her mother. At the same time she felt a dislike for her and a feeling that her mother had never loved her. She said, "One part of me wants so much to stay with her, and the other part of me has to leave her. I'm so divided. I need my mother's love, but somehow I'm very angry with her." By applying a meridian therapy technique* she was able to recall a moment when she silently screamed, "Please let me live! I promise I will never be a burden to you."

Through the healing process that ensued it became clear that her mother, in the early months of pregnancy, had made a decision to have an abortion. She was only stopped from going through with it because her husband insisted that he wanted her to have the baby. Anne reported feeling a great fear that "the opportunity for life" would be lost if her mother went through with the abortion. It was a contract made while she was still in her mother's womb. In her effort to fulfill her side of the bargain, to "never be a burden" if she was allowed to live, as soon as she was able she felt compelled to take responsibility for every aspect of her life so as not to have to depend on her mother for anything.

The mainstream medical conception of consciousness is that it arises out of biology instead of the other way around—that consciousness is the basis of physical reality. This case strongly suggests that since conciousness is at the foundation of life, all sentient life has awareness. Therefore, as Anne confirmed, we can sense danger and feel threatened, even in the womb. Stanislav Grof noted that "the idea that a functioning consciousness could exist in a fetus was in conflict with everything . . . [I] had been taught in medical school."[1]

---

*In this case she used Emotional Freedom Techniques, or EFT, which will be discussed in greater detail in the following sections.

Another of Kenzie's cases supports this idea:

A psychotherapist came to me for help with a deep-seated snake phobia. The phobia was so acute that any snakelike shape—a spiraling bamboo in the corner and even a road winding into the distance—triggered an extremely fearful reaction. Using a meridian therapy technique, it soon became evident that the client had never actually seen a snake let alone had a traumatic experience with one. It turned out that when still in his mother's womb his mother had encountered a large snake in the kitchen. People in the house were screaming, "Look how it curves!" and "Look how fast it is!" Caught up in these reactions, the mother's fear was transferred to the fetus, creating a phobia that, in the mature person, existed with no corresponding experience.

Cases like this demonstrate that a person's memories may well reach back beyond the point of birth. How far that may be, and to what extent their memories are their own, is the object of our inquiry. As professional breathing coaches Jon and Troya Turner, pioneers in holistic psychology and medicine, note, "If I accept that the patterns are mother's emotional-mental patterns, then what I am experiencing during some regression therapies are not actually my own experiences—because I am not wholly me yet—but are my mother's pre-birth and labour feeling patterns."[2]

The power of techniques like Rebirthing Breathwork, used in John's case, arise from the connection between our breath, our "inner energy," and the quality of our awareness. This connection has been recognized and used by shamans, yogis, and mystics for thousands of years. As holistic physician Deepak Chopra observes, "Breath is the junction point between mind, body, and spirit."[3] The form of breathing used in these forms of breathwork is called *circular breathing*. It consists of connecting the inhalation and the exhalation in one smooth circuit while "pulling" the inhalation and then completely relaxing the exhalation so that it takes care of itself. Circular breathing is always preceded by relaxation exercises and accompanied by complete muscular relaxation.

It should never be attempted without experienced supervision or train-ing, since things can get out of hand very quickly. Its main effect is to rapidly increase the level of one's inner energy. This has two effects. First, it activates and—when combined with deep relaxation and acceptance—facilitates the integration of deep-seated emotional issues. Second, it facilitates the onset of a greatly expanded depth and quality of awareness. From this it will be evident that the quality of one's inner energy is fundamental to consciousness, healing, and transformation; and this, in fact, is exactly what ancient yogic traditions confirm.

Let's explore the concept of inner energy so we can understand its connection to consciousness in more detail.

What Is Inner Energy?

Inner energy is also called *vital energy* or *subtle energy*. It is known as *qi* (or *chi*) in Eastern medicine and in yogic and martial arts disciplines. In Eastern traditions qi is always accompanied by consciousness or *li*. Qi and li are thought of as being inseparable. A traditional Eastern meta-phor for this relationship is that of the blind horse and the lame rider. The blind horse (representing qi) has the power to move but lacks direc-tion or agency. Conversely, the lame rider (representing consciousness or li) has vision (a sense of direction or agency), but lacks the ability to move. In other words, consciousness and energy are intimately inter-twined; you cannot have one without the other. This alternative model of consciousness sees it as a universal field rather than the by-product or epiphenomena of neural activity. We need to consider which of these models best explains the cases of healing and transformation recorded throughout this book.

A store of innate qi exists in each sentient being. This energy can be enhanced by energy absorbed from the earth, the air we breathe, and the food we eat. In John's case, breathing and relaxation were sufficient to drive his qi up to such a level that it both surfaced and facilitated the integration of the deep-seated emotional blockage related to his traumatic birth experience. Less well known is the fact that qi can also be drawn down, in a form known as *universal energy*. This provides the energy used in the many forms of hands-on healing that have been practiced for ages. In recent years, hands-on healing has become very popular. One tradition that has fueled this popularity is the Japanese practice of Usui Reiki.* This form of hands-on healing is easy to acquire since it only requires a short initiation process to activate it. Reiki has no intrinsic belief system attached to it and is proven to be highly effective. It is especially effective in situations that conventional medicine is unable to address, as Kenzie's mother demonstrated.

One day I noticed that my seventy-five-year-old mother had a few bruises on her arms and legs. Since she had not had any accidents, I suspected that it could be due to internal bleeding. When she visited the doctor he confirmed that this was the problem. His diagnosis was that the spleen was failing to let go of the platelets that thicken the blood and allow it to clot (thrombocytopenia). The bone marrow was producing blood cells, but the spleen would not release them into the bloodstream. Normally the number of platelets should be between 200,000 and 450,000 per microliter of blood. My mother's count was just 8,000. If she were to cut herself, the blood would not be able to clot and would not stop flowing. At first the doctor tried cortisone. The platelet count increased to 160,000, but then fell back down to 30,000 by the end of the treatment. This was still far too low. She was told to wait since nothing more could be done at this stage. The spleen could not be removed since the thin blood would make any operation problematic, and in any case they did not know whether this procedure would work. At this stage I told my mother to set her mind to get well and to start using first-degree Reiki on herself. She accepted this advice and started to systematically apply Reiki to her spleen every day for a few hours. The

---

*It is called Usui Reiki after its founder, Mikao Usui. His personal search to understanding universal healing energy led him to develop Reiki over a hundred years ago.

monthly platelet count started to increase. First, it went up to 60,000, then to 145,000, and then up again to 195,000. When it reached 195,000, her doctor, the head of the hematology department at the university hospital, became curious. He asked her if she was undergoing some other treatment. She told him about Usui Reiki, about which he showed a lot of interest, telling her, "Whatever you're doing, please continue, it's good for you!" After four to five months of systematic, daily self-treatment, she was completely and permanently healed. A few years later, at a conference at which I was one of the speakers, I told this story and thanked the doctor, mentioning his name because he had been so open-minded and supportive. Somebody in the audience stood up and said, "He is also practicing Reiki now."

Needless to say, despite the existence of scientific research about hands-on healing, neither Reiki nor any other form of hands-on healing is recognized by Western science.[4] In fact, skeptics routinely dismiss the idea as *vitalism,* a term that describes the superstitious attribution of supernatural agency to inanimate matter. In doing so, Western science has overlooked the one essential concept that facilitates an understanding of the nature and scope of consciousness. While mainstream Western science is oblivious to the existence of these energy fields, this is not true for the rest of the world. Research into the nature of qi continues to be undertaken in countries such as China and Japan,[5] where the concept forms an integral part of their cultural traditions and practices, including their mainstream medical practices. Qi flows throughout the body and the major organs via a set of channels called *meridians.* The system of meridians provides the basis for a whole range of healing modalities of which perhaps the best known is the practice of acupuncture. Acupuncture is commonly thought of as an ancient Chinese practice,[6] but as the following account shows, this may be an oversimplification.

In 1991 the frozen body of a man was found encased in ice in the Oetz valley, high on the mountains bordering Italy and Austria.

Carbon dating revealed it to be over five thousand years old. The body had been well preserved because of the cold, dry conditions that had endured there for millennia. Medical examination determined that the man had suffered from a number of health problems, specifically arthritis of the lumbar spine and a digestive disorder. But the most remarkable finding was that the body had some fifteen groups of simple tattoos on it, none of which appeared to have any ritual or ornamental significance. Instead, 80 percent of the fifty-eight tattoos corresponded exactly with the same points used by modern acupuncturists to treat the two conditions that the man had been diagnosed as suffering from.[7] An expert opinion on the placement of the tattoos was sought from one of the main Chinese colleges of traditional medicine. Their specialists concluded that two-thirds of the tattoos had been placed on the primary location used to treat back pain, and the remainder were located on or around points used to treat problems associated with digestion.[8] Apparently, early European healers, like contemporary acupuncturists, shared the same understanding of the energy body and how to work with it to heal and relieve pain. This remarkable convergence of diagnosis and practice in different cultures separated by millennia, and on different sides of the planet, suggests that the same underlying reality was perceived, understood, and managed by our ancient ancestors to alleviate suffering and promote healing.

In the early 1980s experimentation regarding the relationship between the major meridians and physical and emotional problems led to the development of a whole new range of highly effective meridian therapy techniques. Chief among these was Gary Craig's Emotional Freedom Techniques (EFT), which grew out of an earlier technique developed by psychologist Roger Callahan, called Thought Field Therapy. EFT involves remaining focused on a specific mental, emotional, or physical discomfort while tapping a few of the key energy meridians. As the tapping progresses, the level of discomfort starts to fall until it is entirely eliminated. That these easy-to-learn-and-apply techniques are capable of eliminating conditions that defy conventional

Western medicine is proof that their underlying model of energy, consciousness, and healing is both substantially correct and an improvement over existing Western models.

Meridian Therapy Techniques

How do the energy body and negative emotions relate to physical illness and mental disorders, to fears and phobias? To answer this question we need to establish what a negative emotion is. For sure it is a tendency—even in the absence of any immediate or apparent cause—to feel anxious, sad, fearful, or angry, to react negatively in inappropriate ways, and to be subjected to certain recurring negative thoughts or memories. In meridian therapy terms, a negative emotion is, at root, a restriction to the free flow of life-force energy, or qi. Our experience over the last twenty years or so is that simply tapping the meridians is sufficient to completely release even the deepest emotional pain, trauma, and anxiety. Our potential to reshape our own lives and help others as well is, therefore, far more dynamic than many of us imagine. It is, in fact, more dynamic than many of us can even begin to imagine. The following story, as Kenzie relates, illustrates how fears and phobias can be addressed and healed, in most cases quickly and efficiently, using energy techniques such as EFT.

At a company meeting I was invited to give a talk to the management team on health and happiness. To demonstrate the power of the new energy psychology techniques to empower more effective self-management, I asked the audience of a hundred or so managers whether anyone had a problem that they would like to resolve. A woman put her hand up. Her problem was an acute fear of public speaking. Because her fear was so intense she could not speak up, and I had to go to her. She was shaking when I joined her in the audience. I started to tap on the woman's meridian points using the standard Emotional Freedom Techniques (EFT) protocol and asked everyone else in the audience to tap along with the woman, tapping themselves, intending as though they were her. At this point they had received no information or training about the technique. Nevertheless, after just two rounds of tapping, the woman's fear was entirely eliminated, and she was able to come to the front of the room and comfortably address the entire audience.

Fortunately, we are now beginning to see the first serious studies of the effectiveness of meridian therapy techniques. And the experiential and experimental evidence is clear: maintaining a clear and present focus on a specific negative emotion while tapping or otherwise stimulating the major meridians results in its complete and permanent release. When that emotion underpins a physical problem (most back pain, for example), the removal of the underlying negative emotion will cause the physical problem to disappear. The same procedure can mitigate, if not remove, a large percentage of purely physical aches and pains. Over the last thirty years or so, the validity of this process has been proven countless times with every form of negative emotion, including fear, sadness, and anger. Even the most severe and intractable of anxiety disorders, post-traumatic stress disorder, or PTSD, can be effectively treated. Studies involving Vietnam and Iraq war veterans have concluded that "EFT treatment resulted in statistically significant drops in participants' levels of anxiety, depression, posttraumatic stress syndrome, and overall psychological distress"[9] and "after EFT treatment, the group [of veterans] no longer scored positive for PTSD, the severity and breadth of their psychological distress decreased significantly, and most of their gains held over time.[10] A 2013 randomized study of veterans suffering from PTSD saw 70 percent of the EFT group score PTSD negative after just three sessions, while 87 percent scored PTSD negative after just six sessions.[11]

In the context of such an otherwise intractable problem as PTSD, these scores are nothing short of miraculous, far beyond anything achievable through conventional approaches. And yet despite overwhelming evidence for its effectiveness, the technique has been almost completely ignored by conventional science, medicine, psychotherapy, and the mainstream media. Why? Because it simply does not conform to mainstream Western biomedical models of reality. It is also freely available and therefore of little interest to profit-driven Western medicine. Anyone can watch the abundance of online how-to videos on EFT and download a manual for free. It's easy to learn and fun to apply, highly effective, natural, and with no side effects.

In the light of her decades of practical, hands-on experience with meridian therapy, Kenzie found that the drawback with techniques like EFT is that it is necessary to locate, identify, and reconnect with the original emotions. However, when it comes to traumatic events, people are naturally wary of seemingly reliving those painful experiences. Still other meridian-based techniques can cause an uncomfortable build-up of energy in the head so that their use is restricted to a matter of minutes on any given day. To eliminate these kinds of obstacles, Kenzie innovated an approach called Mind Connection Healing (MCH), which empowers the client through the use of a natural technique that functions internally in exactly the same way as when you talk to yourself. Whereas most meridian therapies are based on what could best be described as a kinetic approach, that is, one involving the routinized stimulation (e.g., tapping) of specific meridian points, Kenzie's approach is much more conceptually refined, easier to learn and use, and significantly enhanced in terms of its reach and effectiveness. Let me explain.

MCH is based on a protocol that expresses an intent for healing that is used in conjunction with the energy emitted from one's own hands. This healing intention is permanently installed in the mind of the client as a self-affirmation implanted in a meditative state and thereafter can be used to trigger healing at any time or place.

MCH is sufficient in and of itself to heal mental, physical, and emotional disturbances in any person's energy field. In addition—and this is the important point—it is effective for treating others, even when they are at a distance from oneself, as we shall see in examples from Kenzie's files in subsequent chapters. In other words, by incorporating the healing modality within the field, we can now leverage the field's nonlocal, timeless connectivity to empower people as healers and allow them to perform healing not only on themselves, but on others as well, and in a far more dynamic way. It works on people, events, and animals.

The effectiveness of MCH can be seen in situations involving the "mother wound" and the resulting sense of worthlessness and anger that arises in a small child due to the child's perception of their having been emotionally neglected. This kind of situation can arise due to the physical or emotional absence of the mother at an early age and the child's inability to discern this as the unintended consequences of some other demands on their mother's time.

Kenzie's client, a university professor, came to her for help with her unaccountable, lifelong, and intense anger toward her mother. Whatever her mother did for her made her react angrily, dismissing any demonstration of her mother's love and care and even throwing away any gifts she sent her. Using Mind Connection Healing (MCH), Kenzie prompted the client to ask her unconscious mind what situation had originally caused this reaction. One event came to her. At the age of three her parents had left the house telling her to be good and to not do anything to disturb her grandmother, who was disabled. That night she felt very lonely and afraid and yearned for her mother's love and support. The next morning she struggled to dress herself, looking forward to her mother's appreciation of her efforts. When her parents returned later that day they were both very rundown and had her newborn baby sister with them—which came as a big shock to her. The birth had been a particularly difficult one during which both mother and child had nearly died. Despite this, the parents felt that they had to return home from the hospital because of the grandmother's condition and the fact that the first child was still only three. Because the new baby was doing poorly and consuming all of her mother's time and energy, the client said she came to believe that her mother didn't love her anymore and preferred her newborn sister. Her disappointment, shock, and then growing anger lingered into adulthood. Because Kenzie was using MCH, there was no need to dig up and one-by-one identify all of the historical feelings, sensations, and reactions related to these events. MCH's preinstalled healing intention allowed her mind to completely heal not only her rage, but the guilt she felt for mistreating her mother for the last forty years. Her mother wound was transformed into empathy, and she was finally able to accept all the love flowing from her mother into her heart.

Sometimes a single, well-defined traumatic event may be healed in one session, but other times healing means we must address a variety of issues over a longer period of time. This requires that the client commit to their own healing process. Jessica, a businesswoman aged forty-two, was a participant in Kenzie's MCH training. She was overweight as a result of emotional eating. After the training she enlisted in Kenzie's weight-loss group, where each week a particular theme was addressed, and the participants worked both on themselves as well as providing healing support to one another. Here's Jessica's account of her healing her mother wound:

My mum used to make wonderful pastries. They were very tasty, warm and fresh, and smelled wonderful. When I was nine, whenever I came home from school, there was no one at home because Mum was looking after my aunt, who had had a stroke. It was very lonely at home, but Mum's fresh pastries and bagels were always there for me. Of course I devoured them and then had a long nap until Mum came home. This was the time when I first started to gain weight. I became so accustomed to these tastes that I subsequently sought out everything I could eat that was made with flour and salt—bread, pastries, savory cookies, you name it. I always ate a lot whenever I was on my own. Since then I've wanted to lose weight and to keep to a sensible diet. Sometimes I lost weight, but then I always relapsed into overeating, especially when I felt anxious or angry or unable to deal with some problem. I tried many dietary regimes, none of which worked for me. I recognized that I needed to address my underlying emotional issues around my pastry addiction, so I decided to start with Mind Connection Healing. We explored the effects of my early childhood trauma and separation from Mother, and I recalled that when I was nine I had first felt the urge to eat, so I became aware of the influence that my feelings of loneliness were having on me. As a result I was able to begin using MCH to systematically eliminate the various factors that underpin my addictive behavior—the deep feelings of loneliness, an obligation to wait patiently for her, feelings of helplessness, and the need to repress my worries, my impatience, and my impulse to eat and shut down by going to sleep. Using MCH I implanted a subconscious command to allow the fat to melt away and permit myself to become lean. I realized that I had lost any belief that I could lose weight, so I did MCH to heal my disbelief. As I worked with my initial loneliness and all of the resistance to give up on my pastry friends and the comfort they provided, I realized that I did not derive the same pleasure from pastries, nor did I long for or crave them anymore, and so I started eating much less of them. Every time I experienced some worry or anxiety during the day, or whenever I was confronted by something negative, I employed MCH to clear it. During the workshop it became clear to me that this was not only a question of diet, but rather of choice, of preference. I was under no obligation since I am a grown-up and free to do whatever I like. I could choose to eat less, to eat certain foods or not, and exercise or not. All of this is a question of the choices that I make. I have the power and the freedom to express my feelings, my needs, and assert my boundaries.

By the second and third week using MCH I came to realize that I had been eating too many different kinds of things and far too much, and that this was placing a load on my digestive system. Now I don't need to eat that much or indulge in so much variety. Finally, with the help of MCH, I realized that the first time that I felt very lonely was in fact much earlier—when I was just five years old. My mum had to go abroad for about three months and it was quite a difficult time for me. I stayed with my aunt, which was okay, but we were not that close and I didn't feel safe with her. I felt obliged to do whatever I was told and I was aware that I shouldn't create problems, so I suppressed a lot of things, and it felt like an endless wait for Mum's return. As a result, when I was nine and my aunt had the stroke and Mum wasn't home again, all those old emotions were triggered. That was when I really got to the core of my problems. After I used MCH to clear that initial trauma I started losing weight. It became so easy to deal with stressful events, none of which led to me eating pastries! In fact, I don't even think about eating them now. I'm in the process of moving toward attaining my desired weight and body, and I know I can do it. I've already lost twenty-two pounds!

Joan is a thirty-five-year-old electrical engineer who holds an important role in an international corporation. The following describes her story of how she cleared her allergies, the result of her mother wound, using MCH.

For four years I had strong allergy attacks that lasted around twenty-four hours. They occurred nearly every weekend and always started with intense sneezing. Because of the nasal congestion I couldn't breathe properly and had to rest, and this meant that I lost one day of my weekend. I couldn't understand why this was happening every weekend. I had been to a couple of doctors, and after four years a doctor diagnosed me with nonallergic rhinitis. They wanted to start treating me with cortisone, which I really didn't want nor did I believe the diagnosis. In fact, they said that the underlying reason was probably psychological, and that treatment was outside the scope of their competence. The allergy had no seasonality, nor did it occur in any specific location, and it could flare up after a stressful day just as easily as on a good day. During this period my allergy didn't cause me to miss any important meetings or travel, and I found this to be very strange as it wasn't actually interrupting my work. I knew that like every allergy this was somehow related to my subconscious, but I had no idea what that might be.

I decided to work with Kenzie's MCH technique. When I first started treating myself I had the feeling that I was somehow "in the wrong place" or that "I shouldn't be here." I remembered a time when I was ten and I had to study for an important entrance exam to a good school. Over the weekends my mother made me study. At the same time I was worried about the exam, worried that I wouldn't be able to finish it in time and that I might not pass it. While I knew that I had to use my time efficiently over the weekend, at the same time I wanted to play outside, which made me feel guilty. So wherever I was, I was in the "wrong place" over the weekend. By using MCH I cleared the conflict between using my time efficiently and enjoying myself. I reminded my system that those days were long gone and that I had succeeded in all of my exams. I implanted the belief I am free to do nothing and enjoy my spare time. I finally realized that I was in fact more efficient at work after a long, lazy weekend. The allergic reaction diminished immediately, but was still not completely over, so I did MCH a few more times and it came to me: I was still angry with Mom, who insisted that I study more, even though I had already learned the subjects very well. So when she wanted me to help her with some household chores, I would take out a book and start studying. Here was another conflict: I could have played outside if I had helped her, but out of anger I took my revenge on her instead. So weekends at home triggered my irritation, and the sneezing attacks would then start. Using MCH I treated this irritation and experienced a feeling of empathy for my mother and forgave myself and her. At the final stage of the healing process I started dealing with the itching on the roof of my mouth that was part of my allergic reaction and was connected with my irritation with my mother. I understood that I was angry with my mother because she stopped breastfeeding me by tricking me into being disgusted at the sight of breast milk.

It was a life-changing experience to release my early traumas and my reaction to anything that I subconsciously felt wasn't productive, like taking pleasurable time over the weekend. My allergy was completely healed. I now feel no guilt and no irritation—no sneezing, no congestion, and I now enjoy my time off every weekend.

The importance of techniques such as MCH and EFT, apart from their immense value in empowering people to overcome a vast range of mental, emotional, and physical conditions, is that they clearly illustrate the interdependence of our mental, physical, and emotional health and well-being with our energy system.

These energy techniques have something fundamental to teach us about the nature of reality and consciousness. As for EFT, not only does actually tapping one's own meridians work to alleviate or eliminate all kinds of health issues, imagining or visualizing that you are tapping them also works, as does surrogate tapping, where you visualize that you are someone else and tap yourself on their behalf—even if that person is on the other side of the planet! In the case of MCH, in our mind's eye we imagine that we are connecting to the person who needs the healing and then intend to share the MCH healing intention with them before proceeding with the technique. Kenzie has found this to be very effective in healing animals as well as people.

Let's briefly recount another of Kenzie's cases, in this case, one in which she used EFT for remote healing.

> I received a call from a distraught woman whose young daughter had just been diagnosed with deafness. She was very upset about it and afraid that the condition could worsen. She had no knowledge of the meridian therapies that she might use to help herself. I asked for permission to act as a surrogate for the caller. She was happy to give this. I then applied the standard remote meridian therapy protocol to myself as though I was her. Within a couple of minutes the woman's upset had completely disappeared, even though she was hundreds of miles away.

From the point of view of consensual reality, such claims of healing are beyond anything that most people can possibly imagine, let alone accept. Nevertheless, that is how reality and consciousness are structured. Our approach is neither philosophical nor speculative; it is based on thousands of cases that attest to the truth of these practices, practices that any reader can verify for themselves.

While we think of consciousness as the shifting domain of our own local awareness, in fact it behaves more as though it is a part of a much larger, shared whole in which we all partake and which has distinctively fieldlike properties. This is not a theoretical supposition—it is simply the best way of describing the actual experience of working with these energy techniques.

The Mind-Body Connection

The connection between the energy body and our quality of awareness is a direct one. Is it also a two-way connection? Mindfulness is a form of meditative practice that consists in maintaining a state of present-moment, nonjudgmental awareness. Mindfulness is easy to describe, but experience shows that for most people it is difficult to maintain for any length of time. Like riding a bike, mindfulness practice is a practical skill that is easy to learn but only mastered through regular practice.

Recent research on the effects of mindfulness has been undertaken by Richard Davidson, professor of psychology and psychiatry at the University of Wisconsin–Madison, and a longtime meditator. Davidson has demonstrated greatly reduced levels of stress and increased immune-system functioning using mindfulness meditation.[12] More significantly, Davidson's research has demonstrated that although mindfulness meditation might look like "just doing nothing," the areas of the brain that are activated in clinically depressed and anxious people become much less so when they are meditating, and there is increased activation in the areas associated with happiness and contentment. This shift in neural activity is also associated with the growth (neurogenesis) and development (neuroplasticity) of the neural networks that sustain such positive states.[13] People who practice mindfulness are less deeply impacted by negative events and recover far more quickly when they do occur. In other words, health, happiness, and contentment are outcomes of the cultivation of quietude and acceptance, and these are practical skills that can be refined and developed through practice.

Recent medical research has established the value of mindfulness as an adjunct treatment for a whole range of illnesses. The research underlying these findings is consistent with the findings of the emerging discipline of positive psychology. Positive psychology is the study of happiness and positivity and their effects on human health and well-being. Barbara Fredrickson, professor of psychology at the University of North Carolina, Chapel Hill, where she is the lead researcher at the Positive Emotions and Psychophysiology Lab (PEPLab), says that cultivating positive emotions:

- widens the scope of people's attention, broadens their behavioral repertoires, and increases intuition and creativity
- boosts immune function so that people are less prone to illness, and hastens their recovery if they do become sick
- increases resilience to adversity and promotes happiness and psychological growth
- predicts how long people will live[14]

In other words, positivity—what we do with our minds, and how we choose to think and deploy our awareness from moment to moment—has powerful effects on just about every area of life.

When Do "We" End?

An acquaintance of ours, Stephen, was a professional sportsman. He provided us with the following account of an experience that ended his professional career.

I was having my summer holiday with friends. We drank a lot at a club, and I refused to drive us back to the hotel. But my friend said that he felt sick and begged me to drive. I can only remember that an instant after we entered the main road we had a crash. I recall feeling totally free and completely at peace for the first time in my life as I gazed out across the beautiful landscape. Suddenly I felt a powerful pull, as though I was being removed from the scene of the accident. I found myself looking down on the accident. I saw the wrecked car, bodies lying on the road, and people covering them. I recognized one of the bodies as my own. I remember thinking that my time had not come yet, and that I wanted to return and live the rest of my life. And with that, in a flash, I was back in my body, which was racked with tremendous pain.

In this accident Stephen lost his friends and a promising career. After several operations involving the insertion of steel plates, it took him two years to achieve some degree of physical recovery. Near-death experiences such as this occur when a person experiences clinical death (their heart stops), and after being resuscitated they recall significant events related to their death. Research has shown that between one-third and two-thirds of people who have died and been resuscitated have had a near-death experience. In the case of children, this figure is even higher. Some of the experiences that people typically describe include:

- experiencing positive emotions
- being aware of having died
- meeting with deceased persons
- moving through a tunnel
- visiting a celestial landscape
- having an out-of-body experience
- communicating with light
- observing colors and experiencing a life review

Near-death experiences may also include additional elements such as being greeted by higher beings, becoming aware of or being told that it is not their time to die and that they need to return, and recounting details about events that occurred around them after they have died that, on the basis of commonsense understanding, they could not have known about. Finally, many people who have had these experiences report finding a renewed sense of purpose in life, acknowledging the reality of a spiritual dimension to existence, and overcoming their fear of death.

Many people view these phenomena as hallucinations, but this fails to account for those situations in which detailed information about events that took place around the person after they died is recalled. Out-of-body experiences accompany near-death experiences in around 25 percent of cases, allowing people to witness what's taking place around them after they have died.

Another acquaintance of ours, Mark, a senior management consultant who had at one point made light of our energy work, provided us with the following account of his own near-death experience.

> *After suffering a heart attack I was engulfed in a great light and felt a great sense of peace and lightness. I found myself looking down on a still figure on a bed being rushed through a hospital and then undergoing a medical procedure. I watched as one of the nurses knocked over a tray of instruments that fell and scattered across the floor. A doctor was working on a body. I suddenly recognized it as mine! He applied a defibrillator to my chest. I suddenly felt a big pain, followed by intense tingling in my chest area. I also felt very heavy as I was suddenly encumbered with my body once more. A day or so later I mentioned the incident of the dropped instruments to the doctor, who was surprised that I knew about it. After all, I was dead at the time.*

After his experience Mark went on to become a Reiki teacher. On one occasion he helped a man who had been paralyzed from the neck down regain movement in his arms by using Reiki in distance healing. Such accounts suggest a number of important factors relating to the nature of consciousness and reality:

- We are able to separate our awareness from our bodies.
- In this state we can access information that would not otherwise be accessible to us.

- In many cases death leaves our awareness intact, at least for some period of time following the death of the physical body.

If consciousness were just a by-product of neural activity, as the conventional model says, this would not be possible. That accounts like this are reported in at least a third of near-death experiences demonstrates the continuity of awareness after death and the separability of our awareness from our bodies.

In the next chapter we will continue to extend our exploration of the boundaries of consciousness and selfhood by looking at cases in which the origins of a disturbance or trauma can emerge from beyond the limits of biographical history.

4

Healing Issues beyond Our Timeline

In every culture and in every medical tradition before ours, healing was accomplished by moving energy.

ALBERT SZENT-GYÖRGYI

THE CASES THAT WE HAVE DEALT WITH up till now remain within the range of most people's worldview. What helps us to keep them within the bounds of the familiar is that all of these cases refer to events within the subject's biographical timeline. No matter how outlandish these cases appear to be, we are intellectually reassured by the continuity of the subject's physical presence in this lifetime. Such cases may strain credibility, but they do not necessitate a fundamental readjustment or reset of most people's underlying beliefs. There is, however, a class of cases, regularly encountered in the context of energy healing, for which this reassuring continuity is absent. These cases provide a much more profound challenge to conventional notions of selfhood, consciousness, and reality. In this chapter we will show how healing personal issues can reveal a deepseated causal nexus in events that preceded the subject's conception. To make these points we will once more borrow from Kenzie's case files.

Merged Identities

Although everyone's case is unique, variations on the scenario that follows have occurred many times. The loss of a sibling before one is born can lead to a deep and unconscious guilt—quite literally, survivor's guilt.

Janet is an art teacher in her early thirties, with dark, beautiful eyes and a hesitant voice. She came to me complaining that the meridian therapy that she had learned was not working for her. She needed help, since she had felt depressed all her life, though she had not suffered any major traumas that would account for this. She had been to a number of psychotherapists, had used various antidepressants off and on, and tried a variety of complementary therapies. Nothing had worked for her. I first tested her using kinesiology (muscle testing, a way of questioning the unconscious through observing the body's responses to questions) to check her muscular response to various statements, but I could not even get a positive response to her name. Next, I had her perform an exercise to rebalance her energy. This involved having her touch her right elbow to her left knee and her left elbow to her right knee a number of times. I then tested her once more using kinesiology and she now responded strongly to her name. Testing further with kinesiology showed that she did not accept any kind of healing. To address her resistance, we started clearing the issues around not deserving to live and not accepting love, help, or healing. All of a sudden she was in tears and said, "I don't want to live." When I checked with her it emerged that she had felt suicidal, and ten years before had actually attempted suicide. The reason for this was a deep-seated feeling of guilt that she had experienced all her life, but for no apparent reason that she knew of. I now checked whether she had a sibling who had died before her. Janet confirmed this—her mother had had a miscarriage at four months. "What's that got to do with it?" she asked, to which I replied, "We'll see if it has anything to do with it." We next started clearing issues around the statement "Two years before my birth, my sibling died." After a while it came to her that "my sibling died and I took their right to live." She felt that this was in some way her fault. "It feels like I'm responsible for their death," she said. She experienced a deep sense of guilt and pain because of this. We then worked to clear each of these negative feelings. Toward the end of the treatment, she took a deep breath and smiled. She felt light. Her guilt and pain had gone, and she felt innocent and free. In one session we had cleared her resistance to meridian therapy, her resistance to healing, and ultimately, her resistance to life itself. The reason for her depression was also cleared. Janet's voice changed. She said loudly, "It worked! This is so liberating. Guilt? What a silly idea! Why on earth have I felt guilty?"

Children born after the death of a sibling may feel burdened by a sense of responsibility for the life of the dead child, even if they are completely unaware of the fact that such a fetus or child had existed. This is, of course, completely incredible to anyone stuck in the emergentist view of consciousness, which sees each person isolated within their own biographical history.

Let's take one more of Kenzie's cases to further illustrate this point.

A young man came to me suffering from depression and an eating disorder. He had been in psychotherapy but felt that it was going nowhere, and so he had discontinued it. I learned from his mother that she had lost her first son. He had died at age three, six years before my client was born. When I mentioned this to him he stated that he had no particular feelings about it. But when we started to work with the deeper levels of consciousness using one of the meridian therapy techniques he had an emotional breakthrough. He burst into tears, saying that he felt so sorry and so guilty, that he had no right to be alive when his brother should have lived. This powerful upsurge of feelings came as a complete surprise to him, since he had no prior feelings concerning the loss of this brother long before he was born. We worked through these negative

feelings, eliminating them one by one. At the end of the session he said
that a huge weight had been lifted off him. It was as if he had taken on
a load of sorrow on behalf of his brother.

These cases clearly demonstrate that we are unconsciously connected in atemporal ways to family and ancestral currents that invisibly
influence our health and happiness, sometimes in very negative ways.
But as these cases illustrate, it is possible to isolate and eliminate these
influences and free ourselves from their effects. None of these cases
could be treated by conventional psychotherapy for the simple reason
that there was no obvious trauma or upset underpinning the depression
that these people suffered from. In addition, all of these cases would
be considered impossible according to mainstream conventional understanding, which limits consciousness to a person's biographical history.
But it is precisely for this reason that these cases are so important. They
demonstrate that the conventional understanding of consciousness as
arising from brain activity instead of the other way around is fundamentally mistaken.

Here we have another case that illustrates how the loss of a sibling
before a person's birth has had lingering effects on them. But in this
case the sibling had a different, and rather special relationship with the
subject, as Kenzie explains:

Helen was a young, sharply dressed, attractive, successful corporate
media director. After a fifteen-year relationship she finally married her
partner. Three years later, even though there were no problems in the
relationship, she divorced him. A year and a half later she was in another
happy relationship. After just two years, she left him as well. Helen came
to me complaining that she wasn't happy, she felt depressed, and that
each time she found happiness she couldn't help sabotaging it. In her
youth she had seen many happy, long-term relationships in her family.
She was also afraid of being happy, fearing that it would eventually go
wrong. She had a sibling who had died two years before she was born.

When I asked her about him she said, "I can't talk about him . . . I don't even want to hear his name, and I don't want to deal with that." After I explained to her that the dead sibling may be affecting her in terms of her depression, tension, and her sabotaging her relationships, she agreed to deal with her feelings about him. Just talking about the sibling made her cry. While performing one of the meridian therapy techniques she visualized the boy and talked to him, saying, "You died before me and I'm very sorry for that. I accept you as my brother and into the family. I now let you go to the light." At this she cried even more. In her mind she "heard" him answer, "I had to go so that you could come." This confused both of us. Normally in these situations the sibling will answer to the effect that "it wasn't your fault," and then just go. This invariably liberates the person from the burden of negative feelings that they have been carrying. But because this response was so different, I decided to use kinesiology (muscle testing) to try to understand what had happened by asking questions of the unconscious field of her experience. To the statement, "My sibling died before me, it was his life, I shouldn't have taken it," she tested weak and experienced no feelings of guilt. To the statement, "I was him and I died as a child," she tested very strong and felt the full force of its truth throughout her body. This would be consistent with other past-life death traumas, though in this case she herself had been her own sibling. We then went on to clear the emotional issues related to her sense of loneliness, sorrow, and missing her mother and father. She next used the energy psychology protocol to clear associated feelings using the statements, "In that life I had to die early. I can now leave that life behind. I am so glad that I was able to come to the same, and right, family." With this, the trauma was fully released. "I can be happy now," she said. After this she said that she had never felt better in all her life. In the subsequent days everyone who knew her commented on her positivity and the change that had come over her. One week later she said that her life had changed. She felt a great happiness and much more connected. She called her mother to learn how the boy had died. She learned it was from a respiratory illness,

and that he had to be quarantined and could have no contact with his
father and mother before he died, which accounted for the loneliness
that she had suffered in her current life.

Modern culture and its system of health care remain hobbled by a refusal to recognize the nonlocal, fieldlike nature of consciousness and how our mindstream acts as a carrier for both biographical and non-biographical traumas that are locked into family, ancestral, and past-life memories, resulting in a variety of ailments, as the following case illustrates:

One of Kenzie's clients was a professional civil engineer with an
autoimmune disease for which she was receiving medical treatment.
Kenzie knew from experience that autoimmune disease is often connected
with childhood trauma and the suppression of feelings arising from it. *
The client's suppression of her feelings therefore became Kenzie's main
focus for the session. They conducted the session over the internet,
employing Mind Connection Healing (MCH). Because the session was to
be conducted remotely (normally the client is present so their reactions
are far more evident), and given the client's general lack of emotional and
physical sensitivity, it was going to prove extremely difficult to understand
or test her progress or the intensity of any emotional reactions.

The client expressed her problem as being one of repression
(unconsciously suppressing bad memories and emotions), of not feeling
her body, and of being unable to experience any joy in life. More
specifically, she felt that she wasn't loved enough and couldn't feel
her mother's love for her. I started exploring whether there had been
any particular trauma during her childhood that she could recall. She
reported that at three years of age her mother had had another child,
and that she had been jealous of her. In addition, her mother had been

---

*This topic is explored extensively by Dr. Gabor Maté in his bestselling book *When the Body Says No: Understanding the Stress-Disease Connection.*

away for six months studying in another country when she was six years old, but she could not feel anything in particular around these events. But given that the client couldn't feel anything, this itself suggested that she was repressing her feelings.

We started with the most prominent problem: "I cannot feel any joy. I don't want to go on like this." I then "saw" a scene, a room, including a sofa and a coffee table and a lampshade that emitted dim light next to a wall. I asked my client, "Does this mean anything to you?" She answered that her father used to lie on a couch like that. At this she immediately felt heat and a huge stress in her chest. I too experienced a vibration and heat, and the name Mary came to me. I said, "I'm hearing the name Mary," whereupon my client answered, "That's my grandmother's name," and started crying. Her paternal grandmother had had a very difficult life. She had given birth to a number of children, one of whom had died, and then she herself died from bone cancer at just thirty-nine years of age. My client reported that she felt the pain and sadness of her grandmother and realized that she could not express any of it.

Using Mind Connection Healing, we then released the energy of her grandmother and the lost child and sent it to the light. After that the client reported that she was still experiencing some residual discomfort. We worked on freeing all of the remaining effects surrounding Mary's death, and at this point my client recognized that she herself had been Mary in a previous life. It appeared that the suppression of all of her feelings and not being able to feel any joy was due to the nature of that death. At the end of the session she was able to feel all of her negative and positive emotions as physical sensations in her body, and so we were able to carry on, addressing her problems with her sister's birth and her mother being abroad for six months, all of which were healed. She was able to feel and communicate all of her emotions throughout the sessions and started feeling joy and a new zest for life.

Modern cultures are limited by refusing to acknowledge the reality of the consciousness fields in which these traumas, as well as those of our biographical timeline, are stored. And yet anyone can gain first-hand insight into how these fields operate by simply engaging in one of these related energy therapies. Alternatively, they can simply observe the operation of the healing field by attending, as a participant observer, a few sessions of family constellations therapy. As we will see in the following section, family constellations therapy offers an ideal platform from which to observe how the healing field works.

The Family Nexus and the Ancestral Realm

Family constellations therapy is a unique form of therapy developed by German psychotherapist Bert Hellinger, from an amalgam of family therapy and traditional African healing practices.[1] Like family therapy, it sees the family as the context for understanding personal issues; but unlike conventional therapy, it views this family context as possessing deep roots that reach back into the ancestral past and transmit an influence down to the present day. Although it's been many years now since my first experience with family constellations therapy, I will never forget the impression that first session made on me. I felt, quite literally, as though the scales had dropped from my eyes and I could, for the first time, really "see" and understand the hidden mechanics of living. Kenzie and I had no idea whatsoever about what to expect from the session that we both attended, since we simply went along in order to discover what it was all about.

We found ourselves in a large room with about twenty other people, most of whom we did not know and who, with few exceptions, did not appear to know one another. The therapist asked who would like to work on a specific problem. One man in the group briefly stated his problem, giving very few details. The therapist then invited him to select people from the group to represent key aspects of his issue and position them in a way that intuitively represented the dynamics of the situation. This included selecting someone to represent himself. After placing the representatives, the man was asked to sit on the sideline and observe what was about to take place. Having been selected, I was now standing within the group of people in the middle of the room. Something extraordinary now began to unfold. While remaining fully conscious and self-aware, I became subjected to what I can only describe as an emotional overlay, a strong secondary emotion, mental attitude, and physical posture that had nothing whatsoever to do with me—except, of course, the fact that I was experiencing these sensations, but rather more like an outside observer than a full participant. It was a curious state of being oneself and another person at the same time! As the sessions progressed with other members of the group, we began to realize that these secondary emotions, thoughts, and physical reactions reflected those of each person that we were representing. Moreover, it made no difference whether that person was absent, missing, or long dead. It was with these secondary characteristics that the constellation therapist worked to untangle what in some cases were age-old conflicts involving betrayals, abuse, deception, and indeed all of the sordid twists and turns that constitute ancestral baggage. Another extraordinary thing was that as each conflict was resolved in just the way that this would happen if the actual people were present, through sincere apology and heartfelt forgiveness, the quality of the energy we experienced changed. It became less jagged, less fraught with strong negative emotions, until at last it resolved itself in an atmosphere of harmony and peace.

Although this account describes the mechanics of the family constellations process, it does not touch on the inner life of this profound process. For that we need to turn to a real case. The following account was provided by a close friend, Maureen, and details one of her constellations sessions.

In placing my family members, I had placed the people representing my father and sister together, separate from the people representing my mother and myself. The person who represented my mother stood looking at the floor as if searching for something. The person who represented me was standing next to her, her hands held out as though waiting to receive something. The therapist asked the mother what she was looking for. She said there had to be more babies. The therapist told me that this meant that there were dead babies that needed to be acknowledged, and she started throwing pillows on the floor to represent them. The mother was not satisfied and kept saying "There are more, there are more," but there were already many pillows on the floor. Then suddenly the therapist asked me if any of the babies had been born. My mother had had a baby while we lived in Nigeria, and it had died one day later. The therapist brought someone else to stand before the mother and said, "Here is your daughter. Look at her. See her." I think it was at this point in the session that things turned around for me because the mother said, "I can't look at her because I never saw her." I was shocked. This woman who didn't even know my mother was talking with her mannerisms, saying things the way she would say them, and now she was telling us that she had never seen the baby. It was true. My mother had never seen her last daughter. Then the therapist began to line up women behind the mother, her mother, her grandmother, her great-grandmother, energetically reconstituting the lineage of women in our family on my mother's side. About eight women down the line, she came across the blockage in the female ancestral energy. As I watched, I understood that the fear I had had since the birth of my son, the fear that he was certain to die, was not mine, but energy carried through the women in the family, and I was standing with my arms open to accept it. There and then I decided that I was not going to accept that energy. The therapist put me directly in my own role in the constellation and I refused to accept the fear. A couple of weeks following the session, my fear for my son had almost disappeared.

To anyone attending a constellations session it is quite clear that we are dealing with a field effect. The sensations of energy within the constellation are quite tangible. Once a constellation has been formed, it's as though the feelings and emotional tone related to the people being represented exist timelessly and are reconstituted at that specific time and place by the reenactment of a symbolic structure representing them. So accurate is this representation that if a key member of the field is left out—perhaps they were an unknown participant in the drama—then the field will indicate their absence and their place within the constellation. In other words, the "consciousness slice" of that time and place is interwoven timelessly within a field that continues to exert its influence down through its living descendants. For this reason, Albrecht Mahr, a medical doctor, psychotherapist, and specialist in systems therapy, has called it the "knowing field." Within the constellation we feel this energy in terms of both the overall emotional tone of the constellation and the specific feelings of the person that we are representing. The energy is tangible.

In this context it is worth mentioning that various types of intense energy work can lead to an uncomfortable concentration of energy in the head, more so if you've conducted a number of constellations in a single day. Such a buildup manifests as sensations of fullness or pressure. On occasion it can lead to headaches. We may experience similar difficulties if we have studied or concentrated on something for too long and feel too mentally restless to be able to relax. The reason for this is that due to the natural constriction presented by the neck, any increase in the flow of inner energy circulates much less readily and tends to build up in the head, leading to the sensation of pressure. The standard solution to all such problems is a greatly simplified version of the classic Taoist qigong meditation known as the *lesser microcosmic orbit*. The full meditative practice circulates the energy along the major meridians that run from the top of the head down the front of the body before turning under the base of the spine and ascending back to the top of the head via the spine. The short version of this meditation only uses the meridian that runs down the front of the body. The following steps will clear most sensations of mental restlessness and pressure:

In a relaxed way, place your tongue on the roof of your mouth.

Visualize the activity/fullness/pain in your head as a heavy, slow-moving liquid, like honey.

Visualize it moving down through your head through the tongue, into and down the throat, to the front and center of the chest, and then following the center line down the abdomen, stomach, and into the Hari point, which is just beneath the navel.

Place your hand on this point to retain mental contact with it.

Clear your mind of everything else.

You will need to maintain this meditation for at least ten minutes, after which you will begin to feel relief from any discomfort. You will know that the meditation is complete because the release of energy from the head will leave you feeling mentally light and pleasantly empty. That this technique works so effectively is yet further proof that when we talk of inner energy, energy fields, and morphic or knowing fields, we are describing real energy fields, not metaphorical ones.

One of the more educational aspects of family constellations work is that it sheds light on ageless values. Once each person's discordant feelings are reconciled, the quality of the emotions they have been experiencing changes for the better, and the overall atmosphere becomes more harmonious. In the day-to-day life of the person for whom the constellation was performed, old fears, illnesses, and relationship issues fade away and are replaced by a renewed sense of energy and purpose. Time and again we see cases where healing only becomes possible when some past injustice is forgiven. The knowing field is not, therefore, just a passive carrier of neutral information. It is an ethical field in that it preserves the imprint of injustice until atonement is made, something that requires real, not feigned, repentance and forgiveness. Only when these are forthcoming does the ancestral field undergo a "re-set" and cease to exert a negative affect on the family lineage. I call this essential activity "recoding" the field. When this happens, we experience a perceptible shift in the quality of the energy signaling the commencement of the healing process.

The identification of ethics as a defining characteristic of these extended fields of consciousness is vitally important. The way we behave now has profound ethical implications not only for ourselves and the people we affect, it has profound implications downstream, for our descendants and for their descendants. Given that these fields are ethical (see chapter 8 for a more detailed discussion of the ethical dimensions of the field), the implications of our collective action—as families, communities, societies, and indeed, as a global culture—will resonate through time, affecting the harmony and spiritual evolution of the entire planet. For now we will draw out the implications of such cases for our understanding of healing, energy, and consciousness.

Past Lives

For many years Kenzie has volunteered to run workshops in large organizations using energy psychology. Among the thousands of cases, the following one stands out:

During one of my Emotional Freedom Techniques (EFT) training classes at a large company, one of the participants complained of an acute height phobia. Even standing on a small step triggered intense fear. His wife was a psychiatrist and nothing that they had tried had worked up to this point. Whenever he thought about height his body was stretching out in tension while seated and saying, "my body is in pieces." Instead of tapping the meridians, I started using Tapas Acupressure Technique (TAT). He then experienced intrusive memories with no foundation in this lifetime, of standing on the edge of a tall building as though he had been contemplating suicide. Suddenly he felt himself losing his balance and falling to his death. We continued using TAT until all of his trauma was completely cleared. And with that, his height phobia also completely disappeared. He was then able to approach a window high in the building and look down and subsequently he was able to go up to the top floor and calmly look down the six or seven stories to the car park below. As he descended the stairs I heard him saying, "This simply is not possible. I have had a scientific education, it's simply not possible to have lived before, whatever that might mean—and yet . . . " He would never have countenanced energy techniques, since he was a trained engineer. At this I told him, "So am I. My background is in industrial engineering."

Past lives or "past lives"? While many people will have a problem in accepting past lives as a reality, therapeutically our personal beliefs make no difference; the important point is that we engage with the healing process. A trauma or phobia is real no matter what its cause, or seeming lack of one. Traces of past lives can emerge as key factors in any kind of energy work. Although there is an ongoing debate about the validity of recovered memories, there is little debate about the healing associated with their integration. An important point here is that treating all seeming "memories" as actual memories of things that happened within the current biographical timeline can lead the unsuspecting therapist astray. Memories need not be memories of anything that actually happened in the current lifetime or even memories involving oneself. Unlike the various forms of past-life work or regression therapy, the cases that we come across during the course of energy healing are neither sought out nor induced. They emerge spontaneously as a natural part of a person's healing process. The following story, another of Kenzie's cases, illustrates this point.

Alison, a woman in her early thirties, came to me for help with a relationship problem. An attractive woman with bright eyes, though a bit shy, she had earned a degree in civil engineering and physics. She described her problem as being "stuck in a vicious circle of failed relationships." Apparently, she was always looking for a certain physical type in a partner, one that she described as "having a broad chin and looking handsome." But every person she took up with turned out to be highly problematic, so all of these relationships were doomed from the

*start. I suspected that she was attracted to problematic people in order to
avoid lasting relationships and any possibility of marriage. Although her
last broad-chinned, handsome date did not want to have a relationship
with her, she insisted that it could be made to work somehow. "I'm
hoping that he will change and want to marry me. His looks are exactly
those of the person I want," she said. She also said that she experienced
an intense fear of loneliness, of being without a partner or marriage.*

*Alison started using the meridian therapy techniques as she worked
through these insights, and as she did so her fears began to emerge. The
last fears to come up were "I am afraid of marriage" and "He's going
to leave me." We then started to clear these fears. The problem was
defined as "I'm afraid to get married." As she applied the technique
to herself, she sensed that something very sad had happened, and after
that she didn't want to get married. She couldn't recall any particular
precipitating event but felt very down nevertheless. She started to treat
herself using the statement "All the origins of this problem are healing
now." At this point, in my mind's eye I saw the interior of a small mosque.
It was green inside and full of people praying. But when I told her this
she said that it didn't mean anything to her. When she started to treat
herself using the statement "All the origins of this problem are healing
in all of my past lives," she started crying vehemently. She said she could
"see" herself in a small village, wearing a gown and stirring food in a
kitchen. Now the strange thing about these "memories" is that they bore
no relationship whatsoever to her upbringing, her scientific education, or
her sophisticated life and career in a big city. As she continued with the
protocol, the village woman that she identified with was having very bad
feelings about her husband. She remembered his name, Mehmet, and
could even "see" him. He was handsome and had a broad chin. With
this memory she found herself filled with joy and excitement. But all of a
sudden her mood changed and she felt intense fear. She reported that in
this life in the village they had only been married for a couple of months
before he had to go away to war. Next she "saw" a big crowd of people
coming to the door of her village house to tell her that he had been killed*

along with two other men from the village. Then she saw the same small mosque that I had seen earlier, but with three coffins inside it. At this point she experienced immense sorrow and pain in her neck and back, and then throughout her whole body. We worked through these feelings using another meridian therapy technique to clear them. While doing this she said, "Loneliness is my destiny" and "I can't go on, I'm in too much pain. I want to leave my body, I can't endure this pain!" We then cleared these pains and emotions as well.

After she calmed down she said that even though she did not believe in past lives, she was sure that this was real. It was a past-life trauma carried forward into the day-to-day drama of her relationships in her current life. Next I used kinesiology (muscle testing) to ask some questions about what had happened in and around the funeral. It seemed as though she had died suddenly while at her husband's funeral, and the trauma of these events had become locked in her energy body. After clearing all of her negative thoughts and feelings, we started to work with positive affirmations such as, "That life is over now" and "My new destiny is to have a happy relationship and marriage." I asked her to imagine what it would be like to be in a happy relationship and marriage. She was delighted with the session. She said that it was the first time ever she could imagine herself married. The broad-chinned Mehmet she had been looking for all this time now seemed to be just a distant, blurry memory. She no longer felt anything about him. She related that she now felt a great liberation in her life. Her horizons had opened and she found that she was now able to relate to men in new and more positive ways. In fact, she was introduced to four men within a week and chose one of them.

All of the past-life cases that we have seen have arisen in the context of healing some ongoing problem that appeared to have no basis in the person's biographical timeline. Now while the search for past lives is not something that we specifically aim for in therapy, it does come up in a certain number of cases as a by-product of resolving some acute and persistent personal issue. In such cases the problems experienced in this life are directly associated with traumatic events that appear to have occurred just before death in a previous life. It is as though the trauma of these unresolved issues becomes locked in a person's mindstream and then carried forward from life to life. In most of these cases it is impossible to prove conclusively that a past life is involved. Nevertheless, most of these cases strike you with their vividness and strong sense of real events lying behind them, events that continue to influence people's lives and behavior today, as seen in the following case:

> *A rebirthing breathwork client of mine had had an intense interest in ballet since early in life. When first taken to see a ballet she burst into tears, overwhelmed by the familiarity and intensity of the experience. She had always believed in reincarnation and that in one lifetime she had been a ballerina. We commenced the session, and the client, a regular meditator, was able to access a very high level of internal energy that produced sensations of ecstasy and bliss. All of a sudden the atmosphere changed. It was as though the session was thrown, suddenly and unexpectedly, into an intense tragedy. Her entire being, emotional and physical, appeared to be consumed by the experience of having "lost her leg." After integrating these difficult emotions, she then had a sense of a separate lifetime, of being a ballerina who had just discovered that she had lost her leg in an accident, though how this happened was not clear. At the end of the session she felt uplifted and revitalized. She said that she had always believed in reincarnation, but that now she knew it to be a fact and understood it in a far more profound way. Later research revealed that the famous nineteenth-century German ballerina Adèle Grantzow, selected as the first dancer to play the main role of Swanilda in* Coppélia, *had succumbed to an illness that ultimately led to her leg being amputated and her death in 1877. I am not aware of any other ballerina that these tragic events could refer to.*

The benefit someone seeks and takes away from such sessions is never the satisfaction of idle curiosity. It is the integration of some obscure but problematic aspect of their current, day-to-day life. This integration leads to a deep and positive shift in the person's mental, emotional, and physical life. Recurring situations such as conflicts with authority figures or patterns of negative relationships suddenly end, and they experience a profound transformation and improvement in their quality of life.

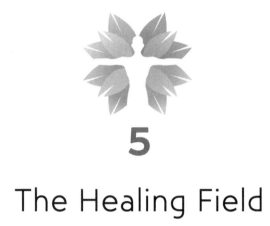

5

The Healing Field

If we break the chain of addiction, violence or other inherited, limiting beliefs, our children and their children and those who follow them are given access to possibilities not available to the ancestors. And thus, the entire lineage evolves.

Dr. Judith Rich

ALTHOUGH THE CASES that we have covered so far constitute only a tiny subset of the thousands of cases that we have dealt with on a daily basis for the last twenty years or so, they are typical. The experiential evidence is clear and unambiguous: A range of biofield energies exists that lie outside those acknowledged by mainstream science. And these fields are deeply implicated in all mental, physical, and emotional health issues and in all effective healing processes.

Disciplines and practices for using these energies underlie the world's many natural healing, martial arts, and spiritual traditions, and they have done so for millennia. Despite this, even the possibility of the existence of such energies is largely ignored by mainstream science. This is due in large part to the common perception that these healing traditions are the products of a scientifically unsophisticated, pre-modern phase of humanity's evolution. On this reading the survival of these ideas into the modern age is only due to the slower pace of development in those countries where such traditions have persisted. Needless to say, this common prejudice against biofield energy healing is only possible if one ignores the available research and extensive body of experiential evidence.

Biofield energies form cocoonlike fields around all life-forms. Somewhat like the phenomenon of blind sight, the ability of the physically blind to sense the properties of objects, these fields are not perceptible to mechanical sense perception but are perceptible to the psychically gifted or as a result of inner cultivation. Disharmony within these fields arises as a result of mental, physical, and emotional trauma and stress. Since these energy fields represent a more fundamental level of existence, healing on this level is disproportionately more effective. What conclusions can we now draw from the cases that we have looked at in the previous chapters?

Our Findings

Our first conclusion is that the healer receives information that is critical to the healing process through empathic engagement. This deeper level of engagement is not just a passive, receptive state of mind, and the insights it gives rise to are not guesswork. It is a dynamic, empathic opening of one's humanity in order to understand and help another person. The healer's empathy is itself an energetic state. To reach out and interact with another person is to shift awareness and energetically interact with their energy field. It is through the medium of this shift that the healer may become aware of information—information that its subject may not be consciously aware of—that proves critical to the healing process. This intuitively derived information has a number of specific attributes:

- It is often represented symbolically or pictorially.
- It may involve "hearing" a name, "seeing" an object, or "smelling" something that is intimately related to a specific traumatic event.

- It may initially appear to be irrelevant, both to the healer and to the client.
- It provides the key that enables a client to reconnect with a past trauma.
- It emerges at just the right time to facilitate the healing process.

The important point here is that this information must be stored or held somewhere. Although it is private information—so private, in fact, that the client may have completely forgotten it or be otherwise unconscious of it—it nevertheless becomes accessible in the context of healing. Because of this, we have little alternative but to suppose that this information resides in an information-bearing field connected with the client. The healer's intention to help is sufficient to facilitate a shift of awareness that allows the unconscious retrieval of information from the client's field. The act of "playing back" that information to the client allows them to remember and reconnect with their feelings about any event underlying their problem. Once this past (distressed) energy state has been activated, energy psychology techniques can then be used to clear the distress. As we noted previously, the efficacy of these energy psychology techniques, even with the most intractable of problems, can be as high as 90 percent.

The healer's intention and desire to facilitate healing provides sufficient navigation, for want of a better word, of the client's consciousness field for the retrieval of relevant information. This is clearly a reversed or goal-governed process. It starts from the goal—the intent to heal—and works to directly retrieve the information that will initiate or facilitate it. This type of goal governed, reverse causation stands in direct opposition to the more usual inductive progress toward discovering something; commonly such insights are called "intuitive," but as a result of their reversing the inductive process we can characterize them as "teleological."

As the scientific method was developed during the sixteenth and subsequent centuries, teleological forms of causation were rejected as contrary to the newly emerging scientific paradigm. Mainstream science is founded on a view of causality based on reductionist materialism, which is to say that all phenomena can be explained in terms of their emergence from interactions between smaller units of matter. From this perspective the existence of abstract "end states" or "goals" that dictate behaviors and outcomes at lower levels is considered unscientific. Although this point of view has been recently challenged by such major figures in the philosophy of science as Thomas Nagel,[1] it nevertheless remains orthodox within mainstream science.

Robust evidence from remote viewing, dowsing, and energy healing points quite clearly to the existence of teleological processes that, given some goal or objective, work backward to retrieve relevant information. In healing work this process depends heavily on the personal qualities of the healer and his or her ability to connect empathically with clients. Such abilities are not, therefore, evenly distributed among a population or readily repeatable, and for this reason they tend to elude formal investigation. Nevertheless, once developed and honed, they work reliably to facilitate healing and integration. Extensive practical experience indicates this teleological faculty stands alongside, and fully equal to, our analytic faculty for discerning material causation. Given the thrust of modernity over the centuries, and specifically its neglect of inner cultivation in favor of instrumentalism, our faculty for direct knowing has been neglected and, ultimately, come to be despised by the dominant and, within its own limited sphere of operation, highly successful reductive materialist worldview.

It is important to stress that these processes do not involve guesswork. Guesswork requires effort. It tends to proceed by placing the available information in some context and trying to work out what the missing parts could be. The spontaneous emergence of information that facilitates the healing process through empathic engagement is quite unlike guesswork.

We will now examine the information and effect-bearing fields within which the healing process takes place.

The Deep Structures of Consciousness

The accounts of healing that we have covered during the previous two chapters entail the existence of a number of layers or strata of integrated information and emotional effects. In most conventional accounts, three to four layers of consciousness are recognized: present-moment awareness, biographical memory, and the biographical unconscious (forgotten and suppressed biographical material). These layers constitute the biographical field of consciousness. Optionally, a collective layer is sometimes recognized. This is the collective unconscious as defined by C. G. Jung. It acts as a repository for the shared archetypal material that recurs throughout human cultural history and is thought of as structuring processes of profound personal transformation. But to account for the experiences associated with the cases that we have been exploring we need to add at least four, and possibly more, fields of consciousness. The existence of these extra layers challenges the mainstream understanding that consciousness arises from neurological activity, instead of the reverse. Two of these extra layers enhance our model of the personal field of consciousness. The other two are collective layers of consciousness. Together I call these fields *the healing field* (or *the healing fields*), since they are regularly implicated in cases of healing, especially once the healer is aware of or attuned to their existence. Many cases of failing to effect healing are attributed to a failure to connect with disturbances held within these fields. The first two (personal) fields within the healing field are:

- **The field of perinatal memory.** This refers to forgotten and suppressed fetal memories during which our experience is, in certain respects, inseparable from that of our mother. It is biographical, its effects constitute a vital part of our identity, but at the same time it is shared with and indistinguishable from our mother's experience. This area has been extensively researched by psychiatrist Stanislav Grof, who has over sixty years of experience researching nonordinary states of consciousness.[2]

- **The field of past-life memory.** This refers to an extended bio-graphical timeline encompassing past lives. This layer manifests as bodily defects and health and relationship issues that can be traced directly to traumatic deaths in previous lifetimes. These cases have been extensively researched by psychiatrist Ian Stevenson and colleagues.[3,4] The emergence of past-life memories is usually associated with past-life regression therapy, but they also tend to surface in the context of a variety of energy healing modalities such as rebirthing breathwork or those involving any of the meridian therapy techniques.

The other two (collective) fields within the healing field are:

- **The field of the family unconscious.** This is an inherited field that affects the members of the immediate family. We have seen that siblings often inherit an unconscious guilt concerning a dead sibling or are burdened with the effort to live a dead sibling's life in addition to their own—even if the sibling died before they were born and they were unaware of their ever having existed. These types of issues typically manifest in the context of the family constellations therapy associated with its originator, Bert Hellinger.[5] They also surface in other forms of energy healing, especially those involving the use of meridian therapy techniques.
- **The field of the ancestral unconscious.** This is another inherited field that affects the members of the extended, multigenerational family. It manifests as emotional, physical, and relationship issues that can be directly traced to unresolved traumas and injustices in the ancestral line. These types of effects typically surface in the context of family constellations therapy.

It is important to note that the idea of these additional fields did not emerge from theoretical or philosophical considerations. They emerged in order to explain recurring cases of healing that hinged on information and traumatic affects from beyond a person's biographical timeline. When these affects were integrated, they triggered the healing of present-day emotional and physical problems that had otherwise persisted through many attempts to deal with them. The existence of these fields, and especially the collective fields, goes far toward confirming the overall fieldlike nature of consciousness and the reality of the extended mind. But unlike the philosopher's concept of the extended mind,[6] which is only extended inasmuch as physical media (diaries and electronic media) can capture information, this idea of the extended mind is the real deal—it is extended in a quite literal sense. Just how far-reaching are these fields? How far does consciousness, and therefore the potential reach of our awareness, extend?

> It occurred to me one day that the earth itself might be a frequency that I could meditate with. So I started to meditate with this in mind and found that I started to experience a state of what can only be described as global or planetary consciousness. This peaceful, harmonious state was quite distinct from the normal meditative states that I was used to.

We can summarize our findings concerning the strata that we have encountered within the wider field of consciousness with a simple diagram depicting the four biographical layers that can be directly aligned with our day-to-day awareness and the two collective layers in which we partake, so to speak, through our wider familial and ancestral connections (see figure 5.1). Please note that I am not claiming that this model is complete; I am merely stating that the existence of these layers has become apparent in the specific healing contexts that we have described in this book. The final point that we want to reaffirm is that these strata of the broader field of consciousness are independently navigable by a complete stranger or group of strangers, as in family constellations therapy. Thus they are emphatically not just "in our heads."

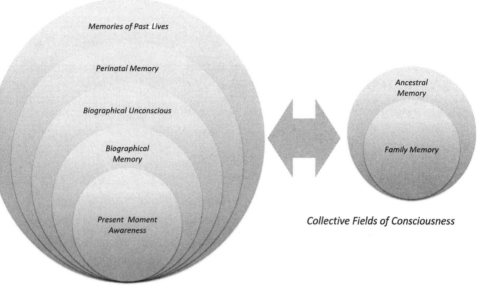

Figure 5.1. The fields of consciousness

The Morphic Field

The second step that we wanted to accomplish was to see if we could find independent confirmation for these ideas. The founder of family constellations therapy, Bert Hellinger, has written, "The first phenomenon . . . is that there is obviously a dimension of awareness that we all share. We all participate in a common field. The representatives often feel and behave like the actual persons they represent."[7]

To better understand this "shared dimension of awareness," Hellinger refers to the work of biologist Rupert Sheldrake.[8] We have already reviewed some of Sheldrake's research in chapter 2. We will now examine the conclusions that can be drawn from this research and how they relate to our own findings.

In biology, *morphogenesis* is the name of the process governing the spatial development and organization of living organisms. The word comes from the combination of the Greek words *morphe*, "form," and *genesis,* "coming into being." Historically there has been a back-and-forth debate concerning the respective merits of genetic versus field explanations of how morphogenesis works. Swimming against the tide of today's mainstream scientific opinion, Rupert Sheldrake has argued that purely genetic explanations fail to explain key aspects of organized growth that can be demonstrated to be field effects.

One of the major problems with Sheldrake's approach is that the nature of the relevant fields is not readily apparent. While it is common knowledge that all living organisms emit a whole range of electromagnetic fields, it is by no means clear whether Sheldrake's morphogenetic fields are electromagnetic in nature or not. In chapter 3 we introduced the concept of vital or subtle energies, energies that are resolutely rejected by mainstream Western science but are the subject of scientific research and mainstream medical practice in the East, where the concept of these energies is culturally normalized.

Sheldrake's morphogenetic fields may also be of this nature. He describes them as "physical in the sense that they are a part of nature, though they are not yet mentioned in physics books."[9] Sheldrake has further extended the concept of morphogenetic fields beyond their immediate biological context to explain the emergence of organized behavior at all levels of life. To distinguish this expanded conception from the narrower biological one, Sheldrake calls these fields *morphic fields* and explains their function as one of organizing "the form, structure, and patterned interactions of systems under their influence—including those of animals, plants, cells, proteins, crystals, brains, and minds."[10]

Sheldrake attributes three fundamental purposes to morphic fields:

- They carry information that provides the environmental input that conditions the development of all living systems.
- They act as a medium of information exchange that coordinates life-forms and facilitates learning even when species are physically isolated from one another.

- They condition behavior and cultural trends and provide a plausible mechanism for such ideas as units of cultural transmission (i.e., memes[11]) or the transmission of values (vMemes[12]).

All of these "top-down" processes are said to occur through a form of causality Sheldrake calls *morphic resonance*. We have all experienced a sense of wonder at the coordination of vast flocks of birds or shoals of fish moving with perfect synchronization at high speed, as though they were of one mind. These displays have the characteristics of being embedded in, and responsive to, a field that unifies and harmonizes their activities. Experiments indicate that whenever a life-form develops a particular quality or ability, all of the other members of that life-form, no matter where they are in the world, develop the same quality or capability in much less time than the first members, despite the fact that they have shared no physical interaction.[13] This form of communication at a distance can only be due to the existence of a shared information-bearing field. These ideas share distinctive parallels, if not identities, with the practical, day-to-day experience of energy healers.

Kenzie's development of Mind Connection Healing (MCH), described in chapter 3, is a good example of how the field can be leveraged to effect healing, regardless of distance, as the following story from her case files illustrates:

I had been invited to teach my method at a maternity clinic and training center. One of the participants, a certified EFT master, was also a midwife. After the first day's training she asked if the method would work for a case of profound grief. I asked her what had happened, and she told me that she had lost her father two months earlier. As I offered my condolences she said, "No, no. I couldn't even feel sad for the loss of my father because my mother is so traumatized by his sudden death. For the last two months she can't even get out of bed and barely eats enough to sustain herself. She has lost contact with everyone. She has been diagnosed with major depression, and nobody has been able to take her out of it; neither the drugs nor EFT have been of any use. We couldn't do anything to help her, and we all feel so helpless. Will your method be able to help?" At this my inner voice said, *Oh my god, this looks very difficult, and then I answered, "Let's give it a try and see if it works."*

A month later I went back to the center to follow up on my previous training and to give another course. She came rushing out with a huge smile and gave me a big hug, thanking me as she exclaimed, "My mom has come back! She has been back to herself for the last two weeks!" I asked her how this had happened and this is how she described the course of the healing process:

"I was in the living room and decided to try to use Mind Connection Healing through the field for distance healing. As you taught us, I intended to connect to her by visualizing a beam of light extending from my heart to her in her bedroom on her behalf. In this way I started to treat her trauma. As I did this I started retching, and as I went on, I could hear my mother also start to retch in her bedroom. Next, she got up and went to the bathroom, where she threw up a couple of times. At that point all of the effects of the trauma were cleared, and my mother came back to life. Since then it has been over three years and she has had no problems with depression whatsoever. It's over. Even with my twenty-odd years of experience with energy psychology, I have never come across such a miraculous case of healing."

Concerning the physical reactions experienced during this particular healing process, it is worth noting that every successful intervention at the level of the energy body always provokes a physiological reaction that acts as a sign that healing has occurred at a fundamental psychoenergetic level. Such reactions can be very muted: a jump or twitch as the meridians clear; yawning or belching are also very common; and the healing of deeper trauma can be signaled by vomiting. These spontaneous physical reactions are entirely natural, very short-lived, and immediately afterward the person will typically feel light, joyful, and relieved, as though a great weight has been lifted off them and their path in life has been cleared of obstacles.

Not only does the field yield enormous healing potential because of its nonlocal characteristics, its atemporal nature allows issues relating to one's upbringing, past lives, and familial and ancestral history to emerge for healing, since the field continues to hold the anger, sadness, and fear that accompanied the original events. These exist as disturbances within the field, and as such they continue to reverberate down to the present day, affecting the health and well-being of new members of the same lineage. Nor is this insight new. One of the earliest references to it occurs in Plato's fourth-century BCE dialogue *Phaedrus,* wherein he matter-of-factly states, "Disease, madness, and great troubles are visited upon certain families through ancient guilt."[14] Such ideas are not among those that conventional thinking would acknowledge or lend credibility to, nor are they among those that most people would feel comfortable voicing in public for fear of ridicule. But that is, nevertheless, exactly what numerous experiences derived from a variety of healing modalities clearly attest to. The problem, then, is in our enculturation and in its foundational concepts (primarily, our notions of selfhood, the nature of consciousness, and the foundations of ethics), which obdurately resist revision even in the face of disconfirming evidence. It is always more comfortable to challenge whether the purported evidence actually is evidence, rather than revising the fundamental categories of how we see the world. The truth is, we are often unaware of the deeply held concepts that stabilize and routinize our experience of reality—until they are challenged by cases from the extreme edges of experience.

Given, then, that disharmony may arise from personal and social injustice, harmony can only be restored when redress has been obtained. We will return to this subject, the ethical nature of these fields, and its implications in chapter 8.

Beyond the Healing Field

Two modern philosophers, reflecting on the implications of Sheldrake's theories, speculate that "if he had confined himself to examining the mores of migrating butterflies or of homing pigeons, he might have encountered less criticism . . . Just how commonsensical is it to believe, for example, that rituals have an existence in some sort of physical sense—a field that is built up by continued activity. Is there, somewhere, a morphic field of Masonic rites?"[15]

Although meant ironically, this is actually an excellent and highly relevant question for us to ponder. Do organizations possessing historical continuity and consistent patterns of ritual practice generate a collective field of memory, ritual, and symbolism? Among magical orders the generation of such fields has always been recognized as one of the necessary prerequisites for achieving magical efficacy and therefore is, in fact, one of the main purposes of ritual activity among both magical and spiritual groups. Such artificial collective fields of shared symbols and energies have traditionally been called *egregores*,[16] an occult concept representing a thoughtform or collective group mind. By undertaking certain shifts in awareness—for example, by partaking in relevant ritual activity or engaging in out-of-body experiences or astral projection—it is possible to "visit" these imaginal realms, these zones existing in a unique space between the imagination and reality.[17] One way to think of them is that they act rather like a blueprint for the realities that they represent, or once represented, in cases where the underlying ritual dynamics are no longer practiced. Access to these subtle planes may occur spontaneously when meditative practice is combined with changes in the level and intensity of our life-force energy. It was such a shift that gave rise to the experiences we recount below.

Our Reiki teacher, Hale, possessed a strong inner energy. Anomalous phenomena often manifested around her. She put this down to the fact that she frequently experienced the rising of kundalini energy. Kundalini *is the name given to the store of life-force energy at the base of the spine. Increasing the level of activation of this energy is the objective of most systems of spiritual yoga. Completely activated, the kundalini gives rise to experiences of enlightened awareness. In the course of rising, kundalini triggers a range of* siddhis, *or psychic powers. I suspect that it was the intensity of Hale's energy that led to the strange visionary experiences recounted here. These experiences occurred during a group meditation that Kenzie and I undertook with her involving seven or eight people. During the meditation, like a vivid dream, I became aware that I was standing in a hall. The floor consisted of black-and-white squares arranged like a chessboard. On the floor to my right lay a coffin, and curiously enough, I saw that I was lying in it. A railway track led past it to the left and entered a dark tunnel. I followed this track and entered the tunnel. As I moved through it, the tunnel bent upward, and I found myself entering a pool of bright light so intense that I couldn't make out any details. It is difficult to express the depth of feeling, the sense of homecoming and acceptance that I experienced there. Afterward, when I shared my experience, I found that Kenzie had also had a near-identical experience—the same checkered floor, coffin, railway line, and tunnel. How could we have shared the same bizarre surroundings in a meditative state? In a subsequent meditative state Kenzie made out some additional features of this strange environment. It contained a lectern from which a long tongue descended like a red carpet being unrolled and a booming voice saying, "A well-hung tongue." This strange expression puzzled both of us. Neither of us had any idea what it meant or referred to, nor is it one that would naturally occur to most English speakers. You can imagine my amazement when some months later, reading a nonfiction book by the novelist Andrew Sinclair, in which he explored the lives of his Templar knight ancestors, who were deeply involved in the origins of Freemasonry, I came across the following obscure lines from the initiation rite of an eighteenth-century Scottish Masonic lodge:*

"Question: Which is the Kye of your Lodge? (translation: what is the key of your lodge?)

"Answer: A well-hung tongue."[18]

Now while this usage can be fairly described as strange, it is even stranger that it should spontaneously occur to someone from a different country and culture with no knowledge of, interest in, or involvement with Masonry. Those who study such things will recognize the checkered floor as characteristic of Masonic lodge rooms worldwide, and the coffin as a recognized symbol of the third-degree or Master Mason, a degree that enacts the symbolic death and resurrection of the candidate.

How could the semisecret imagery and practices of Freemasonry spontaneously occur to people who have no relationship with the order, and certainly not in its more recent eighteenth-century Scottish guise? Given that all of this emerged spontaneously, that it occurred independently among two people with no connection with Masonry across a geographical and cultural divide, and that it involved accurate references to obscure symbolism and ritual phrases, how can we explain it? It would appear that the archetypes of the Masonic lodge room and its rituals, as well as those of other secret societies, exist on a subtler level of reality, one that is accessible via certain altered states. But if such ritual systems exist as morphic fields, do they also possess or exert resonance effects?

This experience was not just a shared visual theater; it was to have a deep and unexpected dynamic. It was connected with a profound shift that I experienced with the nature and quality of my self-perception and understanding, a shift I can only explain as a relativization of my ego-based selfhood in favor of a broader "witnessing" selfhood. The most obvious external marker of this shift was that I freely and easily abandoned my many-years-long enjoyment of tobacco and alcohol. I just felt that I no longer needed them, that they were not healthy, and that I should simply abandon them. If I still wanted these things, the larger "I" that I now had access to simply forbade them; they were not good for my smaller, desiring self. This relativization of the ego has remained to this day, and this is surely the point of the initiation. It enacted this process symbolically by representing the candidate as having died, only to be resurrected, brought back to life, and lifted up to proceed on a higher, that is to say more aware and less instinctively reactive, trajectory in life.

We will pursue this subject further in the next chapter by examining even more extreme anomalous experiences. We will seek to answer the questions: What else does the collective field of consciousness contain? And can other forms of awareness operate within it? Once again, advanced healing practices will turn up some unusual presences.

6

Healing on Extended Plus of Existence

Spirit work is based on the emergence of an intersubjective space where individual differences are melded into one field of feeling and experience shared by healer and sufferer.

JOAN KOSS-CHIOINO

OF ALL THE CHAPTERS of this book, this one is perhaps the most challenging. I want to emphasize that I grew up in a staunchly secular rationalist and humanist tradition. My academic training in analytic philosophy included formal logic, the theory of meaning, and the philosophy of science. It was a rigorous, focused, and entirely, for want of a better word, *grounded* course of study. The conclusions that I have come to in the intervening years and reported here have been forced on me, so to speak, by the sheer weight of thirty-five years of experience with a wide range of energy-based modalities and some twenty years of professional energy healing work. These conclusions go against everything that I had once believed to be true of reality. I report these cases just as they occurred. Some of them are disturbing. All of them pose a significant challenge to our commonsense conception of the borders of selfhood, autonomy, and the underlying nature of reality.

The Bounds of Reality

Most of us think that what we see is all there is. Yet there is ample evidence that what we see is only a small fraction of what exists. That there is a gap between these two becomes apparent when we encounter certain people and entire cultures with fundamentally different perceptions of reality. The respected anthropologist Edith Turner wrote about the conflict she experienced between her scientific training and her actual experience undertaking fieldwork in a traditional society. One day while attending a healing ritual among the Ndembu people of Zambia she distinctly felt a sense of a gathering intensity within the ritual space as the ritual progressed. "I felt the spiritual motion, a tangible feeling of breakthrough going through the whole group," she writes.[1] Watching the healer's hands scrabbling on a woman's back, she reports, "I saw with my own eyes a giant thing emerging out of the flesh of her back. This thing was a large gray blob about six inches across, a deep gray opaque thing emerging as a sphere."[2] She described this object, the revenant of a deceased person, as "a miserable object . . . more akin to a restless ghost . . . There is spirit stuff. There is spirit affliction; it is not a matter of metaphor and symbol, or even psychology."[3]

We may never know for certain, but it would appear that her intense engagement with the ritual process drew Edith Turner into its ritually generated field, allowing her to see, at least for a short time, what was taking place on a deeper level of the healing process. This type of experience is neither rare nor is it confined to the remotest regions of the world. In fact, we find parallel accounts in the ethnographic literature as well as in the day-to-day experiences of many energy healers worldwide. The segregation of these deeper layers of reality from our day-to-day awareness leaves us with a skewed understanding of "what exists" and what forces may be acting on us.

We have already considered the intense fields of familial and ancestral consciousness activated through the ritualized process of family constellations. We have seen how these fields extend to encompass fields generated during the course of ritual healing. Extrapolating from these cases, we can now begin to understand some of the more extreme examples found in the ethnographic literature.

A famous, indeed infamous, example happened to anthropologist Bruce Grindal when he slipped, uninvited, into a Sisala death divination ritual in Ghana. The ritual was undertaken to ascertain the reason for the sudden and unexpected death of the royal drummer. In a 1983 essay, "Into the Heart of Sisala Experience: Witnessing Death Divination," Grindal describes how, as the ritual progressed, he experienced stronger and stronger psycho-physical effects, including intense feelings of terror and dread as well as powerful stomach contractions accompanied by moments of greatly heightened awareness. Suddenly he experienced a great jolt at the base of his skull, as though his head had been severed from his spine. At this, "a terrible and beautiful sight burst upon me. Stretching from the amazingly delicate fingers and mouths of the *goka* (the ritual performers), strands of fibrous light played upon the head, fingers, and toes of the dead man. The corpse, shaken by spasms, then rose to its feet, spinning and dancing in a frenzy . . . The corpse picked up the drumsticks and began to play."[4]

Those experienced with such modalities as kundalini yoga may well recognize Grindal's psychophysical symptoms as connected to the activation of his own latent kundalini energy and therefore understand just how powerful the ritual field generated by the ritualists was. Experiences such as this naturally raise many questions. Did the dead drummer actually rise from the dead, or was the entire scene purely hallucinatory? Would an independent observer have witnessed the scene in the same way, or merely perceived a group of ritual dancers performing obscure movements around a burial pyre? Of his experience Grindal noted that "the canons of empirical research limit reality to that which is verifiable through the consensual validation of rational observers. An understanding of death divination must depart from these canons and assume that reality is relative to one's consciousness of it."[5]

Indeed. Given his enculturation, the unsuspecting anthropologist could hardly have anticipated the impact of attending, albeit uninvited, a ritual process that revealed the psychophysical underpinnings of this African ritual and the changes it engendered in the quality and depth of the perceptions of the observers and participants. Most of us remain completely unaware and unsuspecting of the effects of unseen influences—those of the family, ancestors, past lives, and the deceased—on our health and well-being. These influences may be far more pervasive than many of us suspect, as Kenzie relates:

> I was staying with a friend and student while teaching a training course in her town. We prepared the couch for me to sleep on, but when I lay down I was overcome with an overwhelming sense of heaviness. I felt that someone had died there and that this person had been unaware of the fact that she was dying. I felt a penetrating energy come over me. My student confirmed that everyone who had visited her would be overcome with similar feelings of heaviness and never stayed very long. I started talking to this presence, saying, "You should go to the light. You will find healing there. Now go to the light." We then sent energy to the situation and prayed that whoever it was would realize that they had died, that they were trapped between the worlds, and that they could be healed by making their transition. After a little while the feelings of heaviness released and the atmosphere throughout the house brightened up. I learned later that the neighbor's six-year-old son would never come in my friend's house. He complained that an old lady across the street was continuously staring at him from the window of that room. Returning from the training the next day, the driver recognized the address that we had given him and started to tell us about the old woman who used to live there. He said that she had been bedridden, lying in that room for many years before finally dying there.

The Phenomenon of Haunting

Classic hauntings are usually associated with the lingering attachments of the deceased to certain aspects of their incarnated life. These attachments include places or objects to which they were especially attached or the manner and circumstances of their death. The idea of haunting and what being "deceased" really implies is troublesome in more ways than one. Modern culture has no place for questioning these things or, indeed, anything else that upsets its positivist outlook on what it deems to be reality. And yet year in and year out, across the world, these phenomena continue to be widely encountered and, in some cases, recorded. Although the phenomenon of haunting is extremely elusive, it is nevertheless accessible to the psychically gifted and to those who are able to extend their awareness to encompass these extended planes of existence. The following experience, provided by Amanda, a close friend who is also a manager in a transnational corporation, illustrates just how extensive the phenomena can be in the wake of a major disaster. It also highlights the healing work undertaken by certain esoteric groups:

I had noticed a certain executive at work—we had a nodding acquaintance—though what drew my attention to her I'm really not sure. We finally met thru a common friend and realized we had much in common, with shared interests in spirituality, meditation, and healing. Shortly after the big earthquake in Haiti, she approached me and asked if I wanted to help the people affected by it. I answered that of course I would. She then explained that she was a part of a larger group and that the nature of the help they provided was to assist people who had died suddenly and unexpectedly and were still lingering, lost on the earth plane, trying to make their transition. The help that was envisaged involved projecting myself onto the astral plane, gathering together those lost between the planes, and then bringing them to a certain place where their transition could take place. That night, during my regular meditation, I intended to project to that dimension to help those in need. I found myself in a zone that was not of this earth. There was a lack of light—it was an unearthly greenish gray color—but I could still see. First I saw an old man. He was crying and looked scared and confused. His eyes were red from crying. He didn't know where he was or what had happened to him. He was sitting on the rubble next to a fire. Crying, he asked me where everyone else was. I told him that he was safe. I asked him to wait there for me to come back and that I would bring help. At this stage I had no clue what else to say. As I continued looking for others, I saw another old man holding the hand of a five- or six-year-old boy. It was his grandson. I knew they were both dead, but the old man was still trying to rescue his grandson. My heart sank for them. I told him that he should wait until I came back. Next I saw an old woman. She was still under the rubble—in fact, this was how she perceived her situation. I helped her remove the rubble. I felt that her lungs had collapsed. I helped her sit up, brushed the dust from her clothes, and sent Reiki to her lungs until she felt better. I asked her to wait for me until I came back. The next morning, the first thing I did was to share my experience with my friend. At this point I wasn't even sure if I was making any of this up. I certainly didn't know how to help those people. My friend reassured me that my experience was valid and asked me to go back. She told me to do everything to convince them to come with me, and if necessary, to imagine putting a Red Cross vest on. She then asked me to take them along a path to a park across from a large library building. She told me that this is where the Akashic records are kept. Once there, she asked me to invite the relatives and loved ones of those people to come and assist them in transitioning to the other side. I felt extremely nervous about attempting all of this. I didn't know if it would work or if I could really help them, but I had no choice but to try. That night I returned to the same plane. It wasn't hard to find them. I told them I had good news and that I would take them to where they would be reunited with their families. It wasn't hard to convince them. I visualized the path and found myself across from the library building. Their loved ones came one by one and led them away to the library. The next day when I awoke I was exhausted, completely drained, and I felt very sad. I still wasn't sure if all of this had been a real experience or not. I again shared my experience with my friend, and she said that she had seen me outside the library but that I wasn't ready to see her and the other helpers who had gathered there to assist in completing the process of transition. She explained that they use different methods to convince people to make their transition, including creating an elevator of light or a bridge. She confirmed that I would feel exhausted since I was operating on a plane for which I was not energetically prepared and had fully exposed myself to their emotions. It took me a couple days to regain my energy, but it had been really worth it.

Hauntings are not simple, unitary phenomena; there is no one explanation that covers all cases. Nor can they be understood solely in terms of their external manifestations, including temperature fluctuations, electromagnetic anomalies, and so forth. Hauntings are also profoundly intensional patterns of activity. By *intension,* as distinct from *intention,* I refer to the cluster of concepts based in logic and philosophy around which are our ideas of agency: deciding, intending, acting, and so on, all of which give rise to meaning and, with that, ethical significance. This is a quite different order of understanding, one that cannot be reduced to some corresponding physical description. Classifying hauntings solely in terms of their external manifestations leaves this essential dimension and its underlying significance untouched. It is the business of the healer to be aware of the intensional and ethical dimensions of all phenomena in order to be able to formulate an appropriate response. We can better understand this phenomenon by distinguishing between different manifestations or types of hauntings:

- **Residual hauntings.** Residual hauntings manifest as an extremely narrow band of repeated behaviors, movements, or activities. They demonstrate remarkable consistency, with people reporting similar experiences over long periods of time. They do not respond to or interact with the people who observe them. They behave, rather, like a short video clip that constantly replays. Because of this they are widely understood as a psycho-energetic imprint on the surroundings made while the person was still alive or the related events, such as a battle, were taking place.

- **Disoriented hauntings.** Disoriented hauntings are caused by deceased persons who are either unaware or uncomprehending of the fact that they have died. This can be due to their having experienced a sudden or unexpected death. They may exhibit a strong attachment to the places they were familiar with when alive. They may also experience a strong sense that the living are intruding on their privacy. The account that I gave earlier concerning the old woman and the longer account concerning the earthquake both have elements that fit this category.

- **Petitionary hauntings.** Petitionary hauntings can arise as a result of a deceased person bearing an unfulfilled sense of personal responsibility for resolving some issue. The haunting may involve attempts to contact close friends or relatives who can resolve their unfinished business. Another one of Kenzie's cases illustrates this type of haunting:

I was working on a client's personal issues using energy psychology when all of a sudden I felt something like energy come through me. I experienced a profound sense of sadness that made me feel like crying. Internally I heard the word inheritance. *I asked my client whether there was a problem with an inheritance, and she immediately replied that there was. I had a sense of a person and asked her if this problem was related to a man. Again she replied that it was. I next sensed that there was unfinished business relating to this inheritance, and that the man was saying to my client, "Please, you must take over." My client immediately understood the significance of this exchange. She explained that her uncle had been a prominent lawyer who had helped bring her up. He was like a second father to her, and they trusted each other implicitly. Since he was a respected figure, the family had entrusted their title deeds to him in order to ensure a fair distribution of the lands. Unfortunately, he had died suddenly and unexpectedly before he could fulfill this responsibility. When the family asked for the title deeds, his widow could find no trace of them. With that the matter had remained unresolved for years. Despite the urging of the deceased uncle, my client's first response was that she was afraid to take on such a difficult task.*

Petitionary hauntings can also arise due to a deceased person's sense of injustice. Examples include having their innocence recognized for a crime that they were accused of but that they did not commit, or having someone who stole from them or was responsible for their death recognized as having done so. These hauntings often subside once the issues that concern the deceased person are addressed to their satisfaction.

- **Intercessory hauntings.** These hauntings arise as a result of a deceased person bearing a sense of personal responsibility for protecting or helping some person, usually a close relative. They too subside once the issues that concern the deceased have been addressed. In chapter 2 I gave an example of this type of haunting with Kenzie's case of helping a widow come to terms with her husband's death. In that case, Kenzie once again felt an energy coming through her, picked up the image of a man doing the dishes at a kitchen sink, strong feelings of sadness, and the message, "I don't want you to do this." This message helped Kenzie's client let go of trying to recover the comfort associated with her long, happy, married life; to connect with her feelings concerning her loss; and to resolve the longstanding sadness that had enveloped her since her husband's passing.

Accounts like this challenge us on many different levels. Like the evidence arising from near-death experiences and past lives, they strongly imply the continuity or at least some degree of conscious awareness and a sense of responsibility and ethical judgment beyond physical death. From this standpoint death is revealed to be a transitional state that involves the dissolution, over time, of the relative ego-based personality and its energetic supports in favor of a higher level of identity sometimes called the *soul,* the *mindstream,* or the *higher self* or *overself.*

Traditional systems of spiritual cultivation provide detailed descriptions of this process.[6] Despite the vagueness surrounding the process of dying and the reported sense of unreality associated with the postmortem or intermediate world, what is unquestioned is our ability to undertake healing on such extended planes.

In the context of one-on-one healing, the intercession of deceased persons sometimes forms an inseparable part of the healing process. We have already commented on the advanced retrocausal "navigation" of the atemporal, information-bearing field that the healer's intent brings about. To this we now add its openness to the voices and wishes of the deceased. In the context of healing, this type of communication is always a positive contribution to the healing process. It may also allow for the unexpected reunion with the deceased person, one that reaffirms their love and concern across the boundary of physical death. Such interventions can be a major factor in facilitating healing and closure for the living as well as the dead, of years of pain, separation, and loss.

Spirit/Entity Attachment

Thus far our accounts of interactions with deceased persons have focused on the purposeful phenomena that can arise spontaneously in the course of healing, even when that healing is taking place out of body. In these cases the healer is not deliberately setting out to act as a medium. Once the healing issue (and facilitating the transition of deceased persons is a form of healing) is resolved, any link or communication with the deceased ceases. But unlike these interactions, some attachments can be unwanted and intrusive presences in the lives of people with whom they have no connection, as the following case provided by a close friend of ours illustrates:

I am now fifty-one years old. Two major lifelong problems could have darkened my life forever. Because I chose transformation and healing, it has turned into a totally different journey. When I was a small child there was a period, starting from the age of two or three years of age until I was ten, during which I was sexually abused by my uncle. Later, at fifteen or sixteen years of age, I started drinking to tend the wounds inflicted by this abuse. This turned into a big alcohol problem. In the year 2000 I sought healing for both of these problems. I was able to get help through the use of energy psychology techniques combined with Alcoholics Anonymous. I made good progress, but the alcoholism was difficult to manage and required a lot of self-discipline. During this journey I was introduced to regression therapy. I feel that my healing experience contained such valuable insights that I want to share them with you.

During a session with my regression therapist, after I had entered a trance, my therapist detected the presence of a spirit or entity attachment in my energy field. She was able to determine when it first attached itself to me. At the time of my first experience of sexual abuse I went out of my body to get away from the pain of what was happening to me. The entity had attached itself to me at that time. Up until the regression session, for decades, I had had no idea that I had such an attachment, nor would I have believed in the possibility of such a thing had I been told about it! My therapist was able to enter into a dialogue with the entity, and an interesting story emerged. The spirit or entity had been a prostitute and an alcoholic who had lived in France. She had had a daughter. When her daughter was three years old, the woman was murdered. Because of her sense of responsibility for her daughter she was unable to make her transition and had remained by her daughter's side throughout her life until her daughter died. When I experienced my first sexual abuse and left my body, I was the same age as her daughter when the woman had been murdered. As we noted earlier, it was during this experience that she attached herself to my energy field. The therapist later explained to me that every time these cases appear there is always a positive intention behind the attachment. In this case the entity was trying to help me cope with my emotional pain in the only way that she knew, by using alcohol. After all, she had been an alcoholic herself. It then dawned on me that this helped explain why I had been stealing alcohol from home and always looked for alcohol wherever I went. The therapist convinced the entity to leave my energy field and to seek healing and find peace by making her transition. When I opened my eyes I was amazed by what had happened. Because of the method used, I remembered everything. Nothing had been imposed on me. That night I went to a dinner. I drank a little of the wine that was offered me but found that I couldn't even finish the glass. This was a first for me! Six months have now passed since this healing. I have not had to make an effort to not drink alcohol. I would rate my need for alcohol now at about zero.

We do not claim that every case of addictive behavior is associated with entity or spirit attachment. Addiction is a multilayered and complicated problem. As the work of renowned addiction expert Dr. Gabor Maté underscores, the perinatal nexus—specifically what he calls "maternal deprivation" (where *maternal* refers to a primary caregiver)—provides significant insight into its genesis as well as other Adverse Childhood Experiences (ACEs).[7] Energy psychology techniques can be effective but require a high degree of commitment and collaboration to succeed.

As I emphasized earlier, the cases considered in this book were chosen not because they represent those more frequently encountered, but rather, those that offered the greatest challenges to, and leverage in expanding, our understanding of reality, our place within it, and the potential for positively impacting our own lived experience and that of our family, friends, and community.

If we wish to conceptualize this phenomenon a little more clearly, it is helpful to distinguish between the different parts of the energy body and understand how each is affected by the process of dying. The energy body can be roughly divided between the lower-frequency physical and etheric bodies and the higher-frequency astral bodies and their emotional memories (leaving aside the complex issue of the basis for continuity from life to life and what happens to that). At death, the physical/etheric and astral/emotional bodies separate. The physical body decomposes, and over time its energetic support, the etheric body, also dissolves. The astral body and its emotional charge and memories continue for some time before they too dissolve. On this model, learned experience is transmuted upward to form the basis for the life review and renewed incarnations. In rare cases this natural process can be subverted through the shock of unexpected or sudden death or because of an obsessive attachment to some aspect of incarnated existence. In such cases fragments of the astral body can remain connected to fragments of the etheric body and maintain a discrete existence.[8] Medical doctor and acupuncturist Michael T. Greenwood notes that in the context of acupuncture treatment the practitioner should be prepared for and able to release astro-etheric energy fields, called *Gui*, which attach themselves to a client's energy field: "Since the astral body contains desires and emotions, intense desires that were not transmuted or integrated during life may be released into the universal field, where they can wander or drift about as though looking for a vehicle through which to express themselves."[9]

"Express themselves" in this context means the parasitic attachment to and influence over the behavior of a living being. Such entities can sustain a virtual existence by feeding off the life-force energy of the living. Most people subjected to this form of parasitism do not suspect that their health problems, feelings of lethargy, extreme emotions, or dietary or sexual impulses are being manipulated by an external entity. For one thing, modern culture disdains the notion of such hidden agency, that is, one that remains unseen by the average observer. For this reason the very awareness of this possibility and the skills necessary to discern and deal with it have largely atrophied in modern life. Based on their professional experience, some clinical psychologists[10] and psychiatrists, including Dr. Alan Sanderson of the Royal College of Psychiatrists and Dr. Shakuntala Modi, a transpersonal hypnotherapist practicing in Wheeling, West Virginia, have been led to acknowledge the reality of spirit/entity attachment and understand its impact on mental and physical health. They deal with it through techniques gathered under the rubric *spirit releasement therapy*.[11,12,13] Nevertheless, in general, modernity

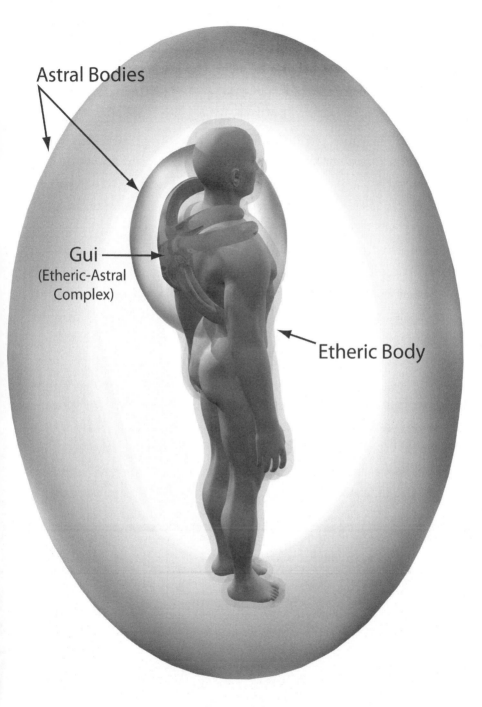

Astral Bodies

Gui
(Etheric-Astral
Complex)

Etheric Body

Figure 6.1. An etheric-astral complex, or *Gui*
(image courtesy of Michael and Richard Greenwood)

remains unwilling to acknowledge such lived realities. Yet such psycho-energetic fragments account for the majority of the spirit/entity attachments known and recognized in every period and culture. As Michael Greenwood notes, "It is probably such etheric-astral complexes that form the basis of discarnate entities known as *Gui* in Chinese Medicine."[14]

Spirit or entity attachment is often signaled by a persistent muscular stiffness, ache or pain, or injuries that do not heal for which there is no medical explanation. It may also be signaled by psychologically unaccountable addictions or compulsive dietary and sexual behavior. It's important to emphasize that this phenomenon is extremely rare. People who suffer from any of these symptoms need to work through routine medical and psychological processes, especially ones that incorporate the new energy psychology techniques, before they start to explore the possibility of spirit or entity attachment. If such attachments are found, most experienced energy healers can remove them.

Spirit attachment occurs most often in situations where people are energetically vulnerable as a result of abuse, illness, injury, or trauma. They can also arise as a result of exposure to extreme situations or places where anomalous phenomena are known to exist. Spirit attachment is especially associated with places where sudden death is common, such as hospitals. People who have recently undergone surgery or suffered an accident that required an operation under anesthesia may experience persistent problems that never seem to clear up. In such cases it is possible, though still very rare, that a remnant of someone who has recently died in such a setting has attached itself to the person's energy body. When people become aware of these attachments they are experienced as intrusive, sometimes behaviorally manipulative, and always parasitic.

Other Forms of Entity Attachment

Let us now examine one of Kenzie's more bizarre cases that falls within this category:

James, a fit, healthy young man who had recently completed his military service, was referred to me for help. He had, quite literally, lost his ability to eat and had lost 33 pounds (15 kg) in just six weeks. He had made the usual round of doctors, but they had been unable to help him. He only contacted me as a last resort. I started by trying to find some event that coincided with the onset of the problem. But after looking in all of the usual places for an emotional upset, shock, or trauma, I could find no reason for his condition. It then occurred to me to try something radically different. Using kinesiology (muscle testing), I asked if he had been the subject of someone's deliberate ill intentions. To my surprise, kinesiology registered a strong confirming response. With this information we started to use one of the standard energy psychology techniques to eliminate the issue. He was then able to feel the blockage in his body. As the healing process progressed, the sensations moved into his hands and fingers. He started shaking them sharply as though trying to throw off something that was clinging to them. He remembered a girl who wanted to marry him whom he had abandoned. She had been sending him messages while he was in the military. All this was taking place in our garden. I noticed that he was shaking his hands toward a particular bush in the middle of the garden. It suddenly occurred to me to tell him to place his hands on the soil and allow the earth to absorb whatever energy was disturbing him. This seemed to work, since the negative sensations in his hands released. More significantly, he was suddenly overcome by hunger. We offered him food, and he consumed everything we placed before him. It turned out that a woman who had been pursuing him for some time but whom he didn't particularly like had to be told that he was not interested in her. It was after this that his problems with eating started. I sensed that the sudden occurrence of a nonhuman entity attachment on an otherwise healthy young man was due to an act of deliberate ill will—in other words, a spell! The young man was delighted with the outcome and wrote a couple of times to thank me for helping him. But for me this successful intervention was about to take an unexpected and highly unpleasant turn. The next day

I was walking Peanut, my cocker spaniel, in the garden. I had just been thinking how fit and healthy he was for his age, when as he trotted past the bush in the middle of the garden, he yelped and fell. He couldn't walk—all of the movement in his back legs was lost and he could only drag himself along with his front legs. Thanks to the massive amounts of energy healing, especially Reiki, and the dedication and commitment of our vet, who used cortisone on the first day followed by homeopathy and auriculotherapy, we were able to help him recover the use of his back legs after three days of treatment. Thankfully, my dog made a full recovery.

Interpreting Phenomena in a Healing Context

Just because we traditionally use words like *spirit, ghost, demon, djinn, angel, deity,* or even the more neutral *entity* to characterize an anomalous experience such as that described here does not mean that we are committed to a supernatural (in the sense of lacking any material base) view of reality. From my own point of view, if a phenomenon can be reasonably categorized as involving a spirit or entity (like the "ghost" stories previously related or the entity that Edith Turner witnessed emerging during a healing dance), then I assume that its material basis, like the 96 percent of the universe that is made of dark energy and dark matter, simply falls outside consensually recognized sensory limits. The existence or otherwise of such entities may make for an interesting debate, but when in the course of routine healing work you are confronted by phenomena strongly suggestive of external agency, the main concern is not which theory best accounts for it, but how to alleviate the client's suffering in a safe and effective way.

At the center of this issue is a critical question: What is the status of the entities that stand at the heart of these phenomena? The concept of unseen entities leaves most of us with a distinct sense of unease, not so much about the possibility of their existence—a creepy enough idea for sure—but rather, the unease of appearing to oneself as well as to others as superstitious, unscientific, and, perhaps, a little gullible. The facts themselves seem to exist in a far more complex space than most commonsense worldviews are capable of encompassing.

Our context is one of healing and in particular, energy healing. All of the cases we have reviewed so far point to the fact that our day-to-day awareness offers only a narrow and partial vantage point from which to survey the broader reality. At the end of the day, what we call reality is as much a construction of our perception, and therefore as much "in our heads" as it is "out there." When we experience a shift of awareness, the dynamic range of our experience also changes, sometimes radically. When this happens, and depending on how radical a shift we have made, reality can become unrecognizable from the point of view of consensual reality. Is this perception of an alternative aspect of reality more or less real than that of our daily lives? From the perspective of the healer it doesn't matter. What matters is the healing process. The dedicated healer follows their intuition, and their empathy guides them to the heart of the matter. That success rates of anything up to or over 90 percent can be achieved by facilitating a client's own use of purely natural (nonpharmacological) approaches is itself proof of their validity.

Phenomena occurring at the very edges of human experience are radically underdetermined; we simply have too little information to frame a proper understanding of them. The truth, Oscar Wilde once remarked, is rarely pure and never simple, and this is certainly true of anomalous phenomena. While there are many aspects that defy rational understanding, the evidence for their validity is too strong for us to dismiss out of hand. As a result, we must extend our cognitive model by integrating far more factors than we usually allow for. Jacques Vallée, a prominent researcher of anomalous phenomena, has proposed a model for their interpretation that employs six simultaneous dimensions or "layers of interpretation":[15]

- **Physical:** displays a physical presence consistent with other physical objects (e.g., passes in front of or behind other objects, reflects light, heat, and so on)

- **Antiphysical:** displays a physical presence inconsistent with those of other physical objects (e.g., abruptly appears or disappears, passes through other physical objects)
- **Psychological:** triggers emotional responses (fear, surprise, altered states of consciousness) and confounds our attempts at sense-making
- **Physiological:** leaves distinct traces that are not attributable to natural causes
- **Psychic:** associated with classic psychic phenomena such as telepathic communication and out-of-body experiences
- **Cultural:** plays into our existing narratives and counternarratives about what is and is not possible

The world of the energy healer occupies a liminal zone, betwixt and between, where anomalous phenomena become the new normal. The model of reality that evolves in an attempt to understand these phenomena is of a complex, multilayered, multidimensional space inhabited by many orders of being. Each of us can make these worlds more transparent by undertaking the transformation of our own psycho-energetic being. We will cover this topic in the next chapter.

7

Healing through Spirit

Evolution is a light illuminating all facts, a curve that all lines must follow.

TEILHARD DE CHARDIN

THE IDEA OF HEALING through spirit can be interpreted in two different ways. We can think of it in terms of the healing that occurs as a result of having a spiritual experience; alternatively, we can think of it as the healing that arises from the intercession of spiritual forces. We will cover both of these interpretations in the course of this chapter.

Peak Experiences

Healing as a result of a spiritual experience can manifest on many different levels: physically, emotionally, mentally, and/or spiritually. Because of the profound nature of such experiences, it's not easy to conceptualize them, let alone put them into words, as the following account, supplied by a close friend, illustrates:

One day I was sitting in the kitchen. It was sometime around ten in the morning. My son was about six months old then. The house was quiet, and we were alone, taking in some quiet time together. He was sitting on my lap, making sounds that babies make, and I leaned back against the wall, gazing out at the sea. Then something happened. For maybe what was a second if that, every boundary disappeared. There was no me, no son, no kitchen, no building, no sea, no sky. Everything blended together, and the only way I can describe this is as a vast nothingness with everything inside. There was nothing as I knew it, but there was everything all at once. It was a second of utter peace, contentment, and of being whole, yet being nothing at the same time. And then it was gone. Like an accordion closing, just as suddenly it disappeared and all the boundaries fell back in place. I was back in the kitchen, my son was on my lap, the sea was out there. Try as hard as I could, I was not able to bring back that feeling again. I have never had the joy of that moment again, and I have a feeling that I'm not supposed to. That moment was there to open a door for me. At the time I wasn't able to see that door. Many years later, I understand what I was taught that day. In fact it was probably something beyond teaching . . . It was an experience, permission to see what it was really all about. I don't understand why I was allowed to see beyond that door, but I am thankful for it.

Reading this account, we have the distinctive sense of someone having a highly significant experience, yet one that remains essentially ineffable. I can now add, having known this person for many years, that she went on to inspire and facilitate thousands of women in achieving healing, self-expression, and personal empowerment, as though the experience described here provided the inspiration and confidence to pursue the decades of positive public work that ensued.

Fresh understanding as to why such experiences are so significant has emerged from recent clinical practice. Psilocybin, the psychoactive ingredient found in certain magic mushrooms, has been given to terminally ill patients suffering from depression and end-of-life anxiety. The subjects described how this hallucinogenic drug allowed them to experience a shift from ego-centered awareness toward a much larger egoless state of consciousness in which their personal problems vanished and they could empathically review their lives and relationships. One of the researchers, Dr. Charles S. Grob, describes how "under the influence of hallucinogens, individuals transcend their primary identification with their bodies and experience ego-free states before the time of their actual physical demise, and return with a new perspective and profound acceptance of the life constant: change."[1] This description could also be applied to the outcome of much spiritual experience. Such experiences are called *peak experiences,* a term coined by Abraham Maslow, one of the thinkers who established the transpersonal movement in psychology.[2]

One of our recurring themes has been the breadth of the average person's exposure to prescient, anomalous, and otherworldly experiences. Peak experiences are no different. Even in highly secular societies, surveys concerning people's spiritual experiences reveal a surprisingly widespread sense of the spiritual. Based upon reliable, nonpartisan surveys of social trends—such as those conducted by Pew Research—a continuing, generational shift from conventional religiosity (among both believers and nonbelievers) and toward acknowledging having had a spiritual experience is clearly evidenced in the U.S.A.[3] Drawing on the work of pioneering psychologist William James[4] and the educator Frederick Happold,[5] philosopher and scholar Douglas Shrader proposes a useful summary of some of the key characteristics of such an experience:[6]

- **Ineffability:** It is difficult to do justice to the experience in ordinary language.
- **Noetic quality:** It provides insights or understanding beyond those accessible to rational thought.
- **Transiency:** It typically lasts for a relatively brief period of time.
- **Passivity:** Although such an experience can be facilitated through processes of profound inner cultivation, its occurrence is normally outside of a person's control.
- **Union of opposites:** It involves an awareness of the oneness of everything.

- **Timelessness:** Time stops; there is no sense of duration.
- **Emptiness of self:** There is a realization that the phenomenal ego is not the real "I," and there is the realization of a deeper and fuller sense of selfhood.

Three other significant features of peak experiences also emerge:

- Peak experiences are often accompanied by the experience of pure, ecstatic joy and love for all existence.
- Not all peak experiences are transient. It is possible, with suitable yogic accomplishment, to stabilize a peak experience or even gain sufficient mastery to attain one at will.
- Even transient peak experiences have lasting effects on one's worldview, way of life, and ethical outlook. Peak experiences are dramatic and compelling, but their real value lies in their effecting an ethical shift in the quality of one's understanding, depth of compassion, and behavior.

While peak experiences are much more common in the overall population than we might expect, in terms of most people's day-to-day lives they remain rare, spontaneous, wholly unexpected, and extremely transient. The instant we recognize that we are having such an experience, our awareness snaps back to its habitual ego-centered focus. If such states are to become anything more than transient, then clearly something more is required. Classically this has involved parallel activity in three main areas:

- **Purification of the psychophysical organism:** This involves both the integration of outstanding mental and emotional issues and the detoxification of the physical body. In some systems (such as the many forms of spiritual yoga) it also covers the opening of the energy channels and the cultivation (refinement and expansion) of the life-force energy.
- **Training the mind through systematic meditative and contemplative practice:** This allows the mind to become accustomed

to remaining in a state of present-moment, nonjudgmental awareness. It also develops the ability to recognize higher states as they unfold without becoming distracted by them.

- **Adopting a practical, service-based orientation to life.** Apart from the inherent merit of such activities, they serve to maintain an appropriate relationship with reality. The discipline of serving others helps to strengthen our capacity for empathy and compassionate action.

The experience of higher states is not the "property" or "accomplishment" of the ego, which will inevitably try to appropriate all spiritual realizations as its own accomplishment. In fact, the logic of spiritual states works the other way around: spiritual realization is the experience that arises when the ego finally gets out of the way. The world's many spiritual traditions contain numerous examples of people who have stabilized their awareness at these higher levels. Drawing on these rich sources, we see that the progress toward realization possesses a definite structure both in terms of the stages and types of experience encountered.

The Five Stages of the Path

Based on her own experience and a comparison with accounts in classic works of mysticism, British poet and mystic Evelyn Underhill proposed a five-stage process that characterizes the movement of awareness toward the experience of higher states.[7] When stripped of their theological language, we arrive at the following, more generic stages on the path:

- **Awakening:** This often includes such existential changes as becoming disenchanted with the limitations of one's life, becoming aware of or suspecting the existence of a higher order of reality, and developing the aspiration to work toward it. This realization can arise in many different ways. Most of us are immersed in the intensity and demands of day-to-day living. And yet from time to time we experience the feeling that there must be much more to life. We may even feel that this life is just a stage in a much larger process, the outlines of which we can barely sense. Others may feel completely disillusioned with all aspects of life and be hungry for some higher purpose or meaning. However the process is triggered, an active quest for greater meaning and sense of purpose and understanding is embarked on.

- **Purgation:** This involves a progressive awareness of one's imperfections, the growth of the motivation necessary for self-improvement, and the determination to master the techniques and practices necessary to achieve this. For many people this is as far as they are able to get, since the effective use of the available techniques and practices demands self-discipline, commitment, and systematic practice. They also require a degree of external supervision. Identifying and then working on our most sensitive issues is never easy, and there are seemingly an infinite number of distractions that allow us to avoid doing so. With supervision and the choice of the most appropriate techniques, however, the chances of success can be greatly increased. Getting rid of your TV and minimizing the time you spend on the internet are essential prerequisites.

- **Illumination.** Prolonged practice leads to episodes of direct awareness of the unitive order underlying all things. These insights might occur quite rarely at first and last for only a short time, but with prolonged practice their frequency and duration increases. Although transitory, these experiences can have a lasting effect. They tend to broaden our awareness and lead us toward a larger conception of life purpose within a much broader understanding of reality.

- **The dark night of the soul:** This phrase is taken from a classic sixteenth-century work of mysticism of that name by Saint John of the Cross.[8] Prolonged and disciplined practice leads to the progressive dissolution or relativization of the ego as awareness starts to break free from the habitual attachments that have moored it in relation to everyday life. This is experienced as a process of dissolution or slow death. For this reason C. G. Jung used the Greek word *nekyia,* the night voyage, to describe the dark night of the soul. In the language of alchemy this corresponds to the *nigredo,* or the blackening stage believed by alchemists to be the first stage of the pathway to the philosopher's stone.

- **Realization or union:** The final stage, realization or union, is composed of several successive levels or depths. It can manifest in many different ways and may be influenced by the symbols and practices of the tradition within which you are practicing. While this model provides a useful framework for thinking about the process of spiritual development, we need to recognize that it is founded on theistic meditative and contemplative practices. The object of practice within theistic traditions is usually described as "union with the deity." Mystic poet and writer Thomas Merton described the experience of mystical union: "Contemplation goes beyond concepts and apprehends God not as a separate object, but as the Reality within our reality, the Being within our being, the life of our life."[9] Other traditions, especially nontheistic ones, may conceptualize the process in more abstract terms, as the following extract from a classical Taoist text shows:

> One bright ray of light hovers over the Dharma universe.
> When both are forgotten, stillness is numinous and empty.
> In the void of the great expanse, the celestial mind shines.
> The waters of the ocean are clear and the moon is reflected in the deep lake. When there is no birth there will be no death.
> Nothing leaves and nothing comes.[10]

It is not easy to make comparisons between such diverse experiences, even though we suspect that they point to the same underlying realization. They remain separated by significant historical and cultural differences, each expressed in its own traditional language and symbolism. Nevertheless, many people feel that at some deeper level humanity accesses a common core of spiritual experience and realization. A useful model that we can use to explore this insight has been proposed by former professor of religion at City University of New York Robert Forman. His model differentiates three progressively deeper levels of realization: the pure consciousness event, the dualistic mystical state, and the unitive mystical state.[11]

- The pure consciousness event (PCE) is a wakeful but contentless (nonintentional) experience. It involves remaining awake and alert while neither thinking nor acting, and emerging with the clear sense of having had "an unbroken continuity of experience."
- The dualistic mystical state (DMS) involves being in touch with our own deepest awareness, experienced as silence, while remaining fully conscious of the external world.
- The unitive mystical state (UMS) describes experiencing one's awareness as inseparable from the totality of all things, as expansive and fieldlike.

The unitive mystical state marks the outer limits or horizon of human awareness. Attempts to describe it are often marked by contradiction and paradox, a typical example being the classical Taoist saying, "The Tao that can be told is not the eternal Tao."[12] Despite the ineffability of these experiences, we do encounter some striking commonalities that transcend time and culture. The experience of seventeenth-century Welsh mystic Henry Vaughan bears direct comparison with that of Maria Sabina, a twentieth-century Mexican shaman. The vision that they describe recurs often enough, and with more or less the same quality and imagery, for it to be called "the vision of the machinery of the universe." In his poem "The World," Henry Vaughan writes,

I saw Eternity the other night,
Like a great ring of pure and endless light,
All calm, as it was bright;
And round beneath it, Time in hours, days, years,
Driv'n by the spheres
Like a vast shadow mov'd; in which the world
And all her train were hurl'd.[13]

Of her experience, Maria Sabina writes, "You see our past and our future, which are there together as a thing already achieved, already happened . . . I knew and saw God: an immense clock that ticks, the spheres that go slowly around, and inside the stars, the earth, the entire universe, the day, the night."[14]

Peak experiences such as these affect us on many different levels. Mentally, they affirm the insight that all sentient life is connected at some deeper level of being. Emotionally, they provide the confidence that arises from knowing that we endure through many lifetimes. Physically, they are accompanied by feelings of ecstatic bliss traceable to shifts in our inner energy. Over the longer term they free us from the self-obsession, fear, and futility of ego-centered awareness. But even taking all of these factors into account, we are still left with an important question: What is it that makes these experiences so culturally significant?

The Evolutionary Unfolding of Consciousness

In cases involving psychic knowing, merged identities, past lives, and family and ancestral healing we can see how all sentient life is immersed in a vast, timeless web of life. We call the portion of this web that is common to experiences of healing and personal transformation *the healing field*. It consists of information and a degree of harmony or disharmony that when experienced through the lens of human awareness renders positive and negative emotional effects, personal meaning, and ethical values.

The lives of individuals, families, and all sentient life-forms are influenced by, and in turn influence, this multilayered field of consciousness, which has variously been called the *collective unconscious* (C. G. Jung), the *morphic field* (Rupert Sheldrake), the *Akashic* or *A-field* (Ervin Laszlo), and the *knowing field* (Albrecht Mahr). In the context of family constellations we have seen how patterns of negative affect, encoded within the field through trauma and injustice, create patterns of disharmony that exert an influence on the health and well-being of subsequent generations. We have also seen how these patterns can be decoded and brought into the light of day through symbolic reenactment, and then recoded to eliminate their negative charge. This process, which we call *ethical reharmonization,* provides us with a context in which to understand the spiritual value of peak experiences. They are important because they recode patterns of negative affect or disturbance as coherence and provide a more compassionate and stable basis for future action. In short, meditative and peak experiences facilitate the co-creation of reality from a broader, more compassionate perspective.

The Range of Meditative Practices

Of his time spent in silent retreat in a monastery, the famous British travel writer Patrick Leigh Fermor wrote, "In . . . seclusion . . . the troubled waters of the mind grow still and clear, and much that is hidden away, and all that clouds it floats to the surface and can be skimmed away; and after a time one reaches a state of peace that is unthought of in the ordinary world."[15]

At the very heart of most of the spiritual paths in which the aforementioned five-stage model is relevant we find the mastery of certain meditative practices. And while the actual practice of meditation means different things to different people, most of us will probably agree that it should lead to the kind of inner peace and quiet described above. In practical terms, meditation covers a wide range of techniques and practices. Some of these have evolved over thousands of years within different traditions and are designed to achieve specific objectives. Within this vast range of practices we can discern at least five basic patterns of meditative practice:

- **Mindfulness meditation** consists of maintaining a state of present-moment, nonjudgmental awareness. Developing skill with mindfulness is a core discipline in many traditions. Mindfulness has proven to have mental and physical benefits as well as developing the nonattachment that is essential for the manifestation and stabilization of higher states of awareness.
- **Single-pointed meditation** consists of maintaining focus on a single point. Commonly used objects include a candle flame, a mandala, or a photograph that has special significance to you. The practice is used to develop concentration.
- **Compassion meditation** is a heart-centered meditation that involves reaching out to all sentient beings and wishing for the alleviation of their suffering.
- **Contemplation** is a form of meditation involving the meditative exploration of a particular topic or question.
- **Yogic meditation** is an advanced practice that involves some combination of meditative stillness, visualization, sound, breathing, and posture and energy work. Yogic meditative practice, along with other forms of excitation, represents an alternative path to spiritual realization and is the subject of what follows.

The five stages of spiritual realization provide a useful model for understanding quietist traditions such as the many forms of monasticism that use contemplative and meditative practice. Quietude involves withdrawing from sensory excitation, embracing quiet and solitary conditions, and developing the ability to still the mind and enter a profound state of inner quiet. This path contrasts with the paths of excitation and energized meditation.

The Energized Path to Realization

Excitation and energized meditation use high levels of inner energy to force the rapid expansion of awareness. Excitation may involve any combination of music, dance, singing, chanting, energized breathing, as well as the use of powerful, mind-expanding substances or entheogens. These practices constitute a form of rapid induction capable of quickly raising the powerful life-force energy or kundalini that is situated at the base of the spine. These types of practices are often encountered in aboriginal ritual, for example, in the healing dance of the Kung people of the Kalahari.

Both the energized path as well as the path of quietude ultimately meet at the highest level of spiritual realization: the unitive mystical state (see figure 7.1).

The extent to which everyone in the Kung community gets involved in the healing dance does much to offset the strangeness that inevitably surrounds these practices. The healing dance starts during daytime, with women sitting in a group and singing, often with their children, while accompanying themselves by clapping. The men join in by commencing a stamping dance around the women. This singing and

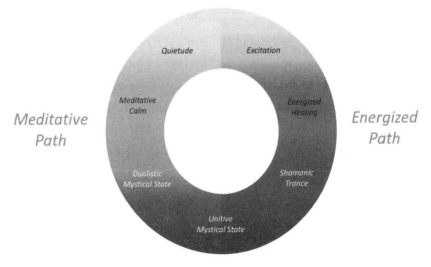

Figure 7.1. The paths of quietude and excitation

dancing continues for many hours far into the night. As it progresses, the rhythm of the dancing intensifies. The dance activates the inner energy of the dancers, which is called *n/um* and is located exactly like its yogic equivalent, kundalini, at the base of the spine.

> N/um, this primary force in the Kung's universe of experience, is at its strongest in the healing dance. . . . The n/um in the healer must be activated for it to become a healing energy. The Kung say the n/um must "gam" or rise up. The singing of songs helps awaken the n/um and awaken[s] the healer's heart . . . The Kung feel that their hearts must awaken or open before they attempt to heal.[16]

As the singing and dancing proceeds, the quality of the energy intensifies. Some people drop out as the energy becomes too intense for them to handle. At a certain point the energy "boils" and rises up the spine to produce a greatly expanded state of awareness called *kia*. In this state the healers can "see" illnesses inside other people's bodies, pull the illnesses out, remote view over great distances, and commune with spirits and gods.

The healing that takes place has three main aspects: "seeing" the underlying causes of mental and physical problems; "pulling out" the illness, depicted as arrows piercing the sick person, either by using the hands or by absorbing the illness into the healer's own body and then expelling it; and interceding with the gods on behalf of the sick person and resisting any spirits or ghosts sent to take the sick person away.

The practices of the Kung healers parallel those of traditional shamans the world over as well as those of certain energy healers. You may recall my own experience with this form of healing described in the first pages of this book. The traditional practices of kundalini yoga and qigong describe similar transmutations of inner energy, experienced as extreme internal heat. These Eastern disciplines are usually practiced on a daily basis for many years. In comparison, the raising of kundalini energy during the healing dance of the Kung occurs in just hours. It is this that accounts for the difficulty, discomfort, and even danger experienced by the participants:

> The training is difficult. Not everyone can stand the excruciating pain of boiling *num,* said to be "hot and painful, just like fire." It makes one cry and writhe in agony. Part of the pain comes from facing one's own death. To heal, one must die and be reborn . . . The terror of *kia* remains despite years of healing, and accepting this recurrent death is the core of the healer's training.[17]

The Yogic Path to Realization

From accounts like that of the healing dance of the Kung it is clear that the path of excitation is not for everyone. The alternative path of energized meditation is typical of the many schools of Indo-Tibetan and Chinese yoga. These traditions use a sophisticated combination of practices, including meditation, postures, diet, breathing, and visualization, combined with quietude to realize the high levels of inner energy that in turn speed the processes of inner purification and refinement. Progress can be accelerated by receiving direct energy transfers from a master practitioner. Such energy transfers can be delivered with different levels of strength, up to and including initiations that trigger peak experiences. It is then up to the practitioner to establish a physical, emotional, and psycho-spiritual foundation capable of stabilizing their awareness at these higher levels. Within the traditions of spiritual yoga the stabilization of enlightened realization is facilitated by the manipulation of the fundamental energies that support and sustain relative awareness. Using techniques such as breath suspension, or *kevala kumbhaka,* these fundamental energetic supports are progressively withdrawn into the central energy channel, the *sushumna,* where they "collapse" on themselves, giving rise to enlightened awareness.[18] This collapse parallels the processes that occurs naturally at death. It is perhaps for this reason that the approach of spiritual realization can be accompanied by feelings of dread. Ultimately, all paths converge in a common experience of spiritual unity. Regardless of the techniques used, the structure of the experience will often exhibit four distinct stages:

- There is a growing dissolution of our sense of selfhood. This is usually accompanied by feelings of fear and dread, as though dying to this world. In mystical traditions this stage is called *the dark night of the soul.*
- At the deepest point of this collapse of our sense of biographical selfhood there is a sudden ecstatic expansion of awareness where all sense of time and place are lost as everything is absorbed in unity.
- Coming down from the ecstasy of union there will be a prolonged period of inner stillness and peace.
- In the days and weeks that follow there will be a gradual resumption of one's habitual connections with reality, though in a uniquely relativized way in that they will simply fail to hold the same addictive and compulsive attraction they once had.

The following account, based on my own experience of kundalini rising, serves to illustrate this sequence:

I sat on a low hill, a still, moonlit swathe of grass ringed by distant trees that stood like a dark enclosure containing reality. My mood plunged with a receding tide of vitality, down, down. I ventured toward the gates of hell, a great gaping darkness, the fear of total engulfment. Patience is the only virtue in such situations, waiting it out and waiting, like an expectant surfer, for the next wave to come. Sure enough, it starts to stir, deep in the base of the spine, at first just the faintest of vibrations that signal "my train's a comin'." The vibrations grow. They grow and expand with the joy of life itself. And then it comes. Unstoppable, pure liquid fire surges up my spine, ecstasy of life, consciousness expands to the four quarters. Bliss beyond bliss. I am all and all is in me. I surf the tides of existence. There is nothing to fear, we always were and always will be. Hours later I return to earth. For days afterward I am at peace and harmony with all of life. I see and feel the beauty of every living thing. As the days pass, I come down. Things start, once more, to bother me. I become a burden to myself. Small irritations trouble me, and I doubt everything, fear the future, and regret the loss of time once more, as though time were finite. But now I can comfort myself. I know and can say that this is all illusion.

This overall process is consistent enough to allow us to depict its main contours (see figure 7.2). The direct paths of excitation and energized meditation are not for everyone. There are significant risks involved in any attempt to force the pace of spiritual development. The dangers are real and take a number of forms. Collectively they are known as *spiritual emergencies.*

Spiritual Emergencies

Stanislav Grof noted the Western tendency to diagnose shifts in our awareness as psychopathological problems rather than as opportunities

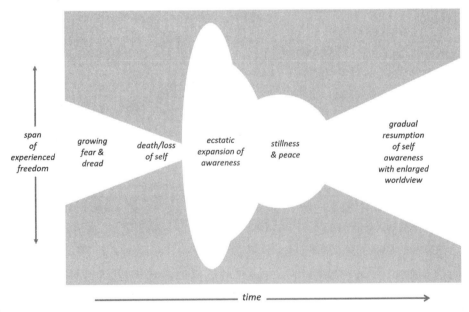

span of experienced freedom

growing fear & dread

death/loss of self

ecstatic expansion of awareness

stillness & peace

gradual resumption of self awareness with enlarged worldview

time

Figure 7.2. The dynamics of spiritual experience

for personal growth and transformation: "There exist spontaneous non-ordinary states that would in the West be seen and treated as psychosis, treated mostly by suppressive medication. But . . . they should really be treated as crises of transformation, or crises of spiritual opening. . . . If properly understood and . . . supported, they are actually conducive to healing and transformation."[19]

By and large, modern industrial and postindustrial societies lack the kinds of informal, knowledgeable, community-based networks that are supportive of such healing and transformation. The preferred approach to the anxiety faced in these societies is to engage in their wholesale suppression by using a broad range of tranquilizers and antidepressants. Few people are well equipped or supported to engage in profound personal or spiritual transformation. For this reason we should not overlook the very real dangers associated with certain practices used to accelerate such changes. This is especially true of the states induced by some of the more extreme practices encountered during shamanic initiation or with the more intense forms of meditation and yoga, especially kundalini yoga.

People undertaking intensive meditative and yogic practices can, as a result of the powerful processes used to purify the psychophysical organism, experience the activation of latent illnesses or the traces of past illnesses as they are flushed from the body. People with a history of mental illness, suffering from unresolved emotional issues or under high levels of stress in their day-to-day life, may experience an intensification of these conditions. If pushed too far, this intensification may become too overwhelming for it to be integrated and may lead to a psychic blowout, which describes the experience of becoming overwhelmed and no longer able to continue with any practice or cope with reality itself.

The adage about making haste slowly applies to all forms of inner work and spiritual development. Perhaps the most important lesson is to not engage in intensive practices, whether it's running a marathon or meditating continuously for a number of days, without first building up your capacity to a level approximating what you are planning to undertake. Following this one simple rule would save many people all manner of mental, physical, and emotional disturbances. Even for a daily meditator, a weeklong intensive is going to be, well, very intense. In this context it is useful to look at the mixture of healing and distress experienced by one regular meditator during a meditation intensive:

> The first day involved intense physical discomfort that arose from maintaining a meditative position for far longer periods than he was used to. Through the next few days the meditator experienced increasingly deeper levels of peace and a broadening quality of awareness until by day five he was able to say, "I experienced bliss"; but by day six he was feeling troubled. "The peace and calm of previous days began to elude me. Thoughts and feelings of conceit, self-consciousness, and judgment surfaced frequently." During a group debriefing session on the final day he reported, "I was overcome by emotion as I tried to speak . . . My eyes welled up with tears, I felt emotionally raw." In conclusion he stated, "Overall, I found the experience healing, self-expanding, calming, rejuvenating, and deeply transpersonal. I experienced stillness, quiet, and self-observation at levels never before encountered."[20]

It is just such an opportunity to experience a profound shift in our awareness that we can take back into our everyday lives and use to improve how we live and interact with others that explains why the path of meditative stillness is so attractive to so many people.

Cases of spiritual emergency demonstrate the extent to which our normal day-to-day awareness is blind to our deeper mental, physical, emotional, and energetic condition. This is one measure of our self-alienation. Intense quietude merely forces us to confront who we really are and what our true condition and posture in life is. In addition to meditative stillness we can use a whole range of techniques to cleanse, purify, and cultivate our inner energy in order to speed up and stabilize the process of transformation. The downside of such practices is an appreciable increase in the risk of mental, physical, and emotional destabilization.

Given the many difficulties, the likelihood of failure, and the very real dangers associated with the path of energized meditation, why, you might well ask, would anyone be bothered to undertake such a journey? There is no easy answer. But I suspect that it emerges from a deep impulse to transcend the limitations of our present condition by moving toward some higher ground with respect to our humanity and to fully realize a hidden but deeply felt potential within ourselves, an upward-moving and expansive impulse inherent in all sentient beings. In short, it is an evolutionary imperative. We will return to this idea in the final part of this book.

Because of the difficulties of attempting a solo ascent of the mystical path, millennia-old traditions have emerged that integrate guidance and direct initiation from an ascending scale of both incarnate and non-incarnate beings. These are traditionally called fully realized teachers, ascended masters, enlightened or higher-order beings, angels, and, ultimately, gods and demigods. Each type of being carries to a greater or lesser degree its own cultural and social baggage, a train of associations that can act more as an obstacle than an aid. One form in which this help materializes is by way of a transmission of energy to the aspirant that triggers varying degrees of peak experience. This process corresponds to the second interpretation that we give to the title of this chapter, "Healing through Spirit." Earlier, in the context of healing on extended planes of existence, we saw that other forms of awareness of varying degrees of sentience also interact with us via shared fields of consciousness. No account of the spiritual path and its effects on the evolution of the fields of consciousness would be complete without considering the higher-order beings that interact via the fields of shared consciousness.

The Transmission of Energy

Many approaches to spiritual development are mediated through a personal connection with higher-order beings. This makes instances of such contact private and worthy of our respect. Short of personal experience, however, this idea may strike many people as extremely dubious if not highly unlikely. One of the problems is that the experiences that underpin these ideas are extremely rare, fall entirely outside mainstream thinking, and are more likely to occur to people who are dedicated to and practicing a specific spiritual path. Nevertheless, wider indications of the validity of such interactions do sometimes occur, as the following events, that I personally experienced, illustrate:

Many years ago I reluctantly accompanied my partner and a few friends to a New Age event. It was a seminar by a popular figure, Tom Kenyon. At the time I had no idea who he was, nor did I have any information about him. In the seminar Tom claimed that he had been contacted during his meditative practice by a group of intergalactic, interdimensional beings he called the Hathors (a name derived from the ancient Egyptian fertility goddess). He stated that these beings exist at a very much higher vibrational rate than ourselves and our day-to-day reality. During the event Tom sought to connect the audience with these beings through his sacred vocal music. This music is inspired by the Hathors and channeled by Tom. As Tom sang, I distinctly "saw," that is to say I psychically registered the presence of many tall columns of light around the stage. These columns seemed to move out and through the audience. One of them appeared to come straight toward me and pass through me. Later on, during the question-and-answer session, a member of the audience asked Tom what these beings looked like. You can imagine my surprise when he described them as "tall columns of light."

The role of higher-order beings is to facilitate the transmission of purifying energies and teachings. Such transmissions form an integral part of all higher rites of spiritual initiation. These rites are quite unlike the rites of passage that effect changes in a person's social status (such as the transition from childhood to adulthood). Instead, the rites of spiritual initiation are voluntary, typically undertaken by only a small number of people, and may, depending on their depth and profundity, involve intensive preparation and purification. They often require the aspirant to take binding vows of secrecy, to abstain from certain behaviors and activities, and to strive to perform certain practices and act in charitable and ethical ways. Finally, they may involve vows of secrecy regarding the initiation process and what is experienced during it. Initiates may form a social group that holds its own private meetings, engages in communal acts of charity, and represents itself as a cohesive force for good in society at large.

One of the most accessible and widely known forms of such initiation is the global practice of Usui Reiki. Reiki is an initiatory, easy-to-use, and highly effective form of hands-on energy healing. Worldwide, all Usui Reiki practitioners can trace their lineage through initiatic transmission from teacher to teacher all the way back to Mikao Usui (1865–1926). Usui was a Tendai Buddhist with an interest in the cultivation of inner energy. He appears to have elaborated the practice of Reiki from a range of preexisting elements and traditions, but the energy itself came to him spontaneously during meditation. It is the continuity of transmission from teacher to teacher that distinguishes authentic Usui Reiki from the many other traditions of hands-on healing therapy that exist today. Some of these are ancient, such as those practiced within the disciplines of qigong or yoga; others are quite recent, such as Therapeutic Touch. Across central Asia and into the Middle East, a range of traditional hands-on healing techniques are known and practiced. Many of these are maintained within ancestral lineages connected to people who were recognized for their spirituality and psychic talents. Contemporary practices such as bioenergy are recognized medical practices in many societies, while a whole range of hand healing practices describe themselves as Reiki, though it would be more accurate to describe them as reikilike, since they have no connection with Usui Reiki and draw from sources of energy unique to themselves.

Whatever the ultimate source of their energy, where all of these energy-based healing traditions meet is at the point of delivery. Their efficacy resides in the generation of an electromagnetic wave pulsing in the extremely low frequency range of 0.5 to 60 Hertz (cycles per second).[21] The difference between healers in terms of their efficacy lies in the fact that an experienced healer may well generate waves of anything up to a thousand times greater amplitude.[22] Reiki's effectiveness is such that it is slowly gaining institutional acceptance both as a research subject and as a component of conventional medical treatment.[23] In recent decades a range of standard medical and restorative devices (pulsed electromagnetic frequency, or PEMF devices) have been designed that generate electromagnetic waves across the same low-range electromagnetic frequencies.

One of the advantages of Reiki is that it is a thoroughly secular practice. It is not necessary to "believe" in Reiki, or anything else for that matter, in order to either provide or receive effective Reiki treatment. Although people have inevitably tended to embed Reiki within their own belief systems, Reiki itself remains independent of any beliefs; it is compatible with all belief systems—or none.

There would be no point in addressing any of these issues if there was not a clear consensus concerning Reiki's effectiveness among its millions of practitioners and recipients worldwide. Whether being used to support greater relaxation, as a preventive measure, or to allay acute conditions, Reiki can aptly be described as a universal panacea. Recall the remarkable case of Kenzie's aged mother, who by using Reiki healed herself of an otherwise intractable condition while under medical supervision so that her week-to-week improvement was monitored by a medical specialist, who was so impressed he went on to become a Reiki practitioner himself!

The world of Reiki is rich in accounts of remarkable healing. Among dedicated Reiki practitioners the explanation is simple. Reiki is a spiritually directed healing energy. Spiritually directed means just that, though the nature of the spiritual direction remains obscure. Modernity, with its positivist "what you see is all there is" outlook, refutes the idea of higher-order beings, even though they have been attested to in every culture since recorded time. Although we think of such beings as supernatural, that is, as lacking a material basis, all that really means is that their material basis, like the 96 percent of the universe made of dark energy and matter, is quite invisible and unknown to us. And yet when we open ourselves to the higher frequencies of love, compassion, and healing, "they"—whoever "they" are—are ready to work with us.

We have been teaching Reiki for over twenty years. Whenever we graduated a new set of Reiki teachers we always celebrated the occasion and inevitably took photographs of the new graduates and their certificates. On one occasion, after summoning the Reiki energy and meditating with it, we took a group photograph of the new graduates in our training room. Kenzie was standing next to them and drew one of the Reiki symbols while she called on the energy to be present with us. This happened just as I was taking the photograph. Something very strange then occurred. I took the photograph using the camera's flash, and as I looked through the viewfinder and clicked the camera, the flash bounced back straight into my eyes. It was as though I had taken a flash photograph directly into a mirror. I blinked and checked the camera as I thought, That was strange, I had better take that again. *I did, and the same thing happened again. Finally, on the third attempt, the camera took the photograph normally. When we uploaded the pictures to the computer, the area around Kenzie, where she had drawn the Reiki symbol in the air, displayed a great circle of light, the inner parts of which had clear three-dimensional properties while its outer edges dissipated outward, blurring the surrounding space in front of the group. Several members of the group had distinctive halos around their heads. There was no mirror or other reflective surface behind the group to account for the flashback from the camera. Whatever manifested in response to being called was real, not imagined, since it had recordable reflective properties. The second photograph had distinct residual effects, while the third photograph was more or less normal.*

The poet Rumi said, "Be watchful—the grace of God appears suddenly. It comes without warning to an open heart." Although transmission can occur spontaneously as *baraka,* divine grace, it is more commonly associated with rites of spiritual initiation specifically

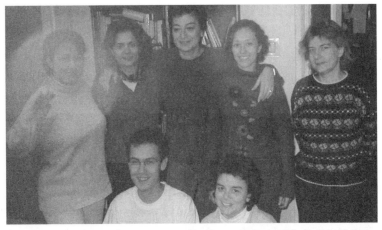

Photograph taken after a group healing session with Reiki. Kenzie is standing on the far left.

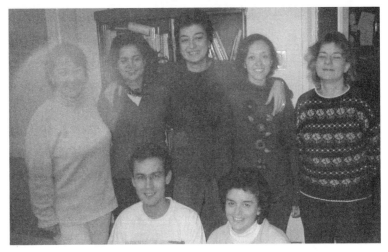

Photograph taken two seconds later

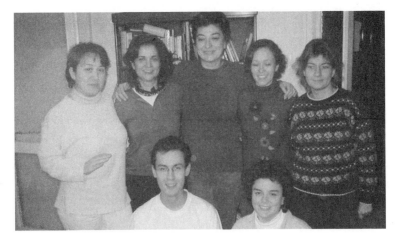

Photograph taken four seconds later

designed to impart this energy. Such rites can be of varying degrees of complexity. For example, they may be accomplished through a simple gesture, such as touching one of the chakras, or with a sacred word or mantra, or even by a look or a thought from a master, as in the yogic practice of *Shaktipat,* which encompasses all of these forms of transmission. In the case of Usui Reiki, the initiation process is a simple procedure requiring just a few gestures on the part of the initiator, during which the initiate simply sits comfortably in meditation. We can think of this form of initiation as entraining the initiate's energy body to the initiator's healing frequency, a healing frequency that they themselves received from their initiator within the Usui lineage. Although this process can be comfortably performed in just ten minutes, the response to it, if any, varies greatly from person to person. As I can personally attest, with proper inner preparation even a simple Reiki initiation can trigger a profoundly spiritual experience:

> *During my Usui Reiki second-degree initiation I experienced entering a bright light. It was of a high intensity but without being in any way harsh or blinding. The sense I had of it was of a higher vibratory state. I could make out very little, but I distinctly sensed the presence of a number of figures within the light. I felt as though they surrounded me and embraced me. I was drowned in a sense of shared unity, acceptance, and love. I stayed as long as I could and then felt myself slowly falling back to normal awareness. As I returned to myself, I was overcome by a great sadness and sense of loss, as though I had fallen from a state of grace, a state of shared and fully realized bliss, back into gross matter. I don't know how long this experience lasted but it must have been for some length of time, for when I "returned," everyone else had finished, and I was left sitting alone.*

In the context of shamanism, the instruction of the shaman is often undertaken by beings connected with his or her ancestral lineage. Similarly, the rites of higher initiation are frequently associated with the intercession of certain beings who maintain a special relationship with the lineage-holders. These are people who have dedicated their lives to preserving the teachings, rituals, and initiation rites. Contemporary examples of such rites are the Indo-Tibetan rites of the higher yoga tantra, known as *deity yoga*. A parallel Tibetan system, Dzogchen, provides a direct initiatory path to the realization of spiritual enlightenment. It is said of this system that it was brought to this planet by a fully realized interdimensional being known as Padmasambhava, who took a human incarnation for this specific purpose. The system he taught and provided initiation into is said to be practiced in thirteen other solar systems.[24] As we noted, the initiations entrain or attune a person or group to various ranges of energies in order to serve a variety of purposes:

- for personal healing and inner purification
- to use the energies to heal others
- to empower others to heal themselves or to initiate others into the energy
- to convey the direct experience of spiritual illumination

The highest spiritual initiations involve the direct transmission of energy from higher-order beings. Such initiations can be delivered one-to-one or simultaneously to hundreds of thousands of people at a time, with no dilution or diminution of effect. Initiations involving intense states of direct spiritual realization are typical of the highest yoga tantra. Similar rites, known as "the Mysteries," were often attributed to ancient Egypt. They were conducted in the name of a specific deity and were found throughout the ancient Greco-Roman world for millennia until they were suppressed by a series of Roman emperors commencing with Theodosius I in the late fourth century CE. Speaking of their initiation into the Eleusinian Mysteries during the first century BCE, a friend of the Roman statesman Cicero wrote, "Nothing is better than those mysteries. For by means of them we have been civilized . . . we have learned from them the fundamentals of life and have grasped the basis not only for living with joy but also for dying with a better hope."[25]

One of the main claims made for the importance of the Mysteries was that they sustained civilization itself. They were thought of as holding "the entire human race together."[26] Why this should be so becomes clearer when we consider the role of spiritual initiation rites in the life of a traditional community. One rite in particular is worth considering, that of the Bwiti religion of West Africa. Briefly, the practitioners of Bwiti conduct a rite that reinforces the ties holding their community together, strengthens their relationship with the ancestral spirits and spirits of the natural world, and provides a direct experience of the divine. The rite extends over three days, involves the whole community at certain stages, and employs a powerful entheogen, *Tabernanthe iboga*.

The Bwiti initiation rite follows the traditional three-stage process that characterizes most rites of passage: separation, liminality, and reintegration.[27] The middle stage of the rite is designed to morally purify the candidate in order to prepare them to meet the powerful spirits of the natural world. This is accomplished by triggering a process of recalling all of the significant events of their life up to that point. The important feature of this recalling is that these events are remembered not from the ordinary self-centered perspective, but from the perspective of the people most affected by them. People who have undergone the rite have testified to its powerful impact on their moral outlook. It civilizes the "raw" components of the personality by making us acutely aware of the consequences of our actions on other people.

Regarding sacred initiation rites, the view of modern classical scholarship is that "the gap between pure observation and the experience of those involved in the real proceedings remains unbridgeable."[28] It is only unbridgeable to the extent that we refrain from undergoing the necessary purification and transformation of our own being and fail to seek out contemporary contexts in which valid initiation still confers an experience of the numinous. As we have seen throughout the course of this book, the walls separating the sacred from the profane, the mundane from the numinous, are never too distant for us to reach, nor too high for us to overcome.

8

Conclusions

Want the change. Be inspired by the flame where everything shines as it disappears.

RAINER MARIA RILKE

Most of us think that what we see is all there is. Yet there is ample evidence that what we see is only a tiny fraction of what there is. Our day-to-day awareness is like a torch that illuminates only a small circle of light in the surrounding darkness. The vaster reality remains invisible to us. It vibrates at frequencies beyond the range of normal perception, much like dark matter and dark energy, about which we know nothing whatsoever.

Since time immemorial people have engaged in practices that allow them to shift their awareness so as to take in more of the hidden reality around them. Such practices have formed an integral part of every human culture from the earliest times to the present day. The broader view they reveal is one in which we are able to shift our awareness within the many strata of consciousness. As we do so, what we experience, what we think of as reality, bends and flexes to accommodate our different perspectives. The fields of consciousness embrace all sentient beings in all times.

What Have These Experiences Shown Us?

From the outset we have focused on some of the most unusual and anomalous experiences imaginable. We took this approach in order to challenge conventional thinking about consciousness and reality and to reveal the much broader expanse of the human spirit. Although many of the experiences covered here are extremely rare in the context of a modern lifestyle, they are widely known and acknowledged within the contexts of energy healing, shamanism, and mysticism.

In chapter 2, which discusses psi in the context of consciousness, we saw that our awareness routinely operates nonlocally. People pick up information about the past, about hidden, distant, and future events with which they have no connection. Conventional thinking, which sees consciousness as a by-product of neurochemistry, cannot explain this and therefore falls back on denying that such experiences are possible. Nevertheless, many of us access such information on an almost daily basis. The ability to shift our awareness—for example, through empathic engagement with other life-forms—helps us relate to the larger community of sentient life-forms, leading us to a greatly enhanced understanding and the possibility of achieving a greater level of harmony and balance with our environment.

In chapter 3, which takes a look at healing within our biological timeline, we saw how energy psychology and meridian-based techniques facilitate healing across a broad range of problems. Some of these problems, such as posttraumatic stress disorder (PTSD), cannot be healed by mainstream medicine. We also saw how the use of energy techniques reveals aspects of our biographical history that require a reconsideration of the limits of consciousness and the boundaries of personal identity. Among these we find memories from our time in the womb. If awareness is produced by the brain as conventional thinking goes, then our timeline should only start in the final month before birth, when there is enough brain for awareness to arise. What we actually find, however, is that people possess memories that relate to all stages of their fetal life, including some memories that are shared with their mother. At the other end of our biographical timeline we saw that our awareness does not end with death. Numerous near-death experiences have been recorded in which people can recall events they witnessed after they were clinically dead.

In chapter 4 we continued to explore the hidden influences that affect our health and well-being outside our biographical timeline. These include such cases as merged identities, where siblings take on the responsibility for the life experience of deceased siblings who died before they themselves were even conceived. In the context of family constellations therapy we saw that our health and sense of well-being may be profoundly influenced by patterns of events inherited from our family and even from remote ancestors who died long ago. In constellations therapy the emotional tone, the people involved, and their individual characteristics become the emergent mental, emotional, and physical properties of the people representing them. This fact raises a fundamental question as to how and where this information and its distinctive emotional charge is stored. Our answer is that it is stored in the larger field of consciousness, since it could not be stored in some complete stranger's brain or DNA. Constellations therapy is only explicable in terms of an unbounded, timeless field of consciousness with nonlocal properties. It also raises a major question as to how our awareness is capable of decoding this field and restoring the responses of people we never knew and who, in any case, may be long dead. Finally, we explored the phenomena of past lives and saw how many successful cases of healing may be associated with clearing the trauma of dying in a previous life.

In chapter 5, which takes a closer look at the healing field, we considered the implications of cases involving psi and energy-based healing covered in the previous chapters. We concluded that these were only possible because consciousness possesses nonlocal, fieldlike characteristics. This tallies with Rupert Sheldrake's experiments demonstrating the existence of an information-bearing and propagating field connected with all sentient life-forms that he dubs the *morphic field*. In the context of healing we find that people's health and well-being is affected by negative emotional states connected with unresolved family, ancestral, and past-life affects that continue to be propagated via morphic resonance. Because they are implicated in a majority of cases involving healing and personal transformation, we call them *the healing field*. They constitute, and are parts of, larger fields of consciousness with which all sentient life-forms interact.

In the context of healing, the past, in the words of William Faulkner, "is never dead, it's not even past"—though it's better to say it's never truly past until something has been forgiven or restitution has been made. This connects the operation of the field to broader issues of agency, meaning, and values. Memory is never neutral; each memory carries a distinctive emotional charge that encodes a distinctive orientation with respect to core values such as justice/injustice, honesty/dishonesty, loyalty/disloyalty, and so on. In other words, the field is also an ethical field.

Ancestral and family memories stored within the field directly impinge on us, whether we are aware of them or not. Just as our awareness is capable of coding and decoding the field's informational and emotional content, a range of healing modalities demonstrate that it is also possible to recode the field and restore its harmony. Recoding the field involves resolving specific conflicts, injustices, and traumas, just as if the people involved were alive and present. This is achieved through a mixture of symbolic reenactment and the reestablishment of harmony between the parties involved, even if long dead. Harmony is reestablished by acknowledging wrongdoing and forgiving transgressions. As a result, operating within the field from a healing perspective has a distinct and ineradicable ethical character. Harmony is associated with such fundamental ethical qualities as justice and respect, and disharmony with the opposite qualities. All of this strongly supports the ancient idea that the field of consciousness, the extended mind, is at root a fundamentally ethical field; and it is within our power to recode the field to create ethical congruence and restore harmony.

In chapter 6, which delves into the bounds of reality to look at spirits and entities, we highlighted the existence of interactions with a broad range of nonhuman beings of varying degrees of sentience. These entities usually exist in frequency ranges that are invisible to us. They can interact with us positively as well as in ways that undermine our mental, physical, and emotional health. On a positive note we explored a range of ghostly phenomena that actually facilitated reconciliation and healing. We also noted that some forms of entity or spirit attachment are positively intentioned. Traumatic experiences can open the energy body to create a point of ingress that allows entities to attach themselves to it. Such entities are not necessarily hostile. They may identify with that person's problems and seek to help by influencing the person's thoughts and behavior. Although contacts with otherworldly lifestreams can provide instruction and help with healing, when these encounters spill over into the lives of ordinary people, their effects can be deeply disturbing. There is no reason for anyone to feel oppressed by any of these realities. Sufferers can take practical steps to cleanse themselves by eliminating the negative emotions and traumas that provide fertile ground for entity attachment.

In chapter 7, we encountered that ultimate expansion of awareness, the spiritual or peak experience. At this level of awareness the innately ethical nature of global consciousness becomes self-evident. To have a peak experience is to embrace all sentient life with compassion and love. Although such a state can occur spontaneously, we seldom have the tranquillity and psychophysical preparedness to sustain it. We identified two paths by which systematic work toward their stabilization can be undertaken: the path of pure meditative contemplation, and the energized path of excitation or energized meditation. The highest mystical states appear to mark the outer limits of human awareness; they represent the furthest extent to which our awareness can stretch. By focusing on such states simply as another experience to be had, we risk missing their real significance. These higher states act as drivers in the evolutionary unfolding of our innate spiritual potential and contribute to the healing and harmonization of the larger web of life. In seeking to realize such states we are following an evolutionary imperative inherent within the nature of the morphic fields that underlie all sentient life.

Realization implies the dissolution of the limited boundaries of selfhood, boundaries that both define us and our perception of the broader reality. How we experience this dissolution varies greatly from person to person, but it is always intrinsically challenging. It is, after all, a foretaste of death itself. All too often, discussions of realization attempt to understand it from a purely experiential perspective. What did it feel like? What did you see? This orientation risks missing the essential point of these experiences. Realization is not just a change in perception; it is a change or shift in our entire psycho-energetic and ethical being. It fundamentally changes how we relate to others, to life, and to the reality of death. It shifts our perception of reality from one mediated by the intellect to one mediated by the intelligence of the heart. Without this evolutionary shift, peak experiences can be gone just as quickly as they came, leaving regret over their transience, a sense of unworthiness at our inability to sustain or recapture them, and a longing for the vision of reality revealed in that one brief moment of realization.

Both excitation and energized mysticism seek to cultivate very high levels of inner energy as the primary vehicle for realizing greatly expanded states of awareness. Needless to say, these practices present certain risks and should not be undertaken casually. Because of the fundamental nature of the shifts involved, we urge caution for anyone seeking to explore these highly energized levels of awareness. They should remember to make haste slowly, to prepare thoroughly, and find experienced supervision. Above all else, balance internal yoga with selfless service in one's community. What these states add to our understanding is a level of comprehension of the larger web of life and our place within it, allowing us to overcome the fears and doubts that are otherwise the lot of the vast majority of humanity.

Consciousness, Evolution, and Values

In Freiburg in 2008 a meeting of experts from the most diverse fields—philosophy, psychology, neuroscience, theoretical physics and theology—was convened to initiate a cross-disciplinary dialogue on the subject of consciousness and spirituality. The forum sought to establish what a model of consciousness would look like that is both true to modern scientific knowledge and to the phenomena reported by the spiritual traditions.[1] The answers that emerged were encapsulated in four main points:

- Consciousness is a fundamental element of reality, like an additional dimension.
- Consciousness is mediated by the brain, not produced by it.
- Consciousness is independent of brain processes.
- Our ability to connect with that which is larger may be a normal state of human beings.

As we have already noted, Sheldrake's concept of the morphic field, Laszlo's A-field, and Mahr's knowing field are all consistent with these views. By acknowledging the essential convergence of these models we can continue to expand and clarify a more complete understanding of the fields of consciousness. Physicist Amit Goswami has usefully summarized Sheldrake's ideas in terms of three defining aspects:[2]

- **Teleology:** By whichever name it is called—the morphic, Akashic, knowing, or healing field—it is a purpose-driven system. It seeks harmony and therefore ethical congruence.
- **Nonlocality:** Because the same template serves all of the life-forms that share its structural properties, it is universally available. In other words, the field is accessible everywhere. This is most evident in the context of therapies like family constellations, where complete strangers are unconsciously able to access and reflect, while retaining full self-awareness, the behavior, thoughts,

and emotions of individuals involved in family and ancestral conflicts, despite the fact that they have no prior knowledge of the people or issues involved.

- **Downward causation:** Through a process Sheldrake calls *morphic resonance,* the field propagates its effects to all of its members.

To these points we can now add the following characteristics:

- The field of consciousness (whether on the personal, family, or ancestral level) is sensitive to the harmony and disharmony that arises in connection with the ethical quality of our actions.
- That emotional disharmony persists in a multigenerational way and is capable of impacting our health and well-being confirms the contention that consciousness must be a pervasive morphic field.
- The field is coded, decoded, and recoded, and therefore (ethically) reharmonized, using defocalized awareness, symbolic enactment, and ethical rebalancing. This itself is astonishing, and brings a different perspective to discussions of consciousness and reality.

The introduction of ethical considerations points to the larger role of ethical behavior in the evolutionary unfolding of all sentient life. Simply put, harmonious action, expressed through such positive qualities as fairness, justice, loyalty, freedom, and respect, equals health, healing, and spiritual growth. Disharmonious action, based on the opposite qualities, halts or even reverses this. We noted the civilizing function of the higher initiations, such as those associated with the Bwiti religion and the Eleusinian Mysteries. These rites were designed to facilitate a shift in awareness that enabled the initiates to view themselves, their communities, and all sentient life as integral parts of the web of life. The result of this experience of the essential unity and continuity of all life is a greatly expanded understanding, tolerance, and compassion. Such shifts fundamentally affect a permanent relativization of the egoic self and allow us to occupy a higher ground with respect to our shared humanity.

These levels of realization represent an upward-moving, expansive impulse that is inherent in all sentient beings. When stabilized, such awareness facilitates higher orders of behavior that manifest evolutionarily higher orders of values. Values are an inherent aspect of both human and animal behavior. As we will see, their manifestation in different societies and cultures demonstrates a deep and consistent structure.

Values

In recent years a leading moral and political philosopher, Alistair MacIntyre, has claimed, "We have—very largely, if not entirely—lost our comprehension, both theoretical and practical, of morality."[3] However we interpret this, it certainly appears as though we face a crisis of values. If nothing else, globalization has led to a collision of cultures, beliefs, and values. But long before the era of globalization, from the eighteenth century onward, modernity experienced its own crisis of values. Ethics has not fared well among modernist intellectual elites. On the one hand, moral judgments have been declared to be no more than random sounds of personal approval or disapproval (emotivism). On the other, various thinkers and philosophers, from Jeremy Bentham (1748–1832) to Ayn Rand (1905–1982), have treated values as systems for the rational optimization of benefits, whether for the larger community (Bentham's utilitarianism) or for one's own private ends (Rand's egoism). These abstract, intellectual conceptions are quite removed from lived experience. At root, values are something that we feel in our innermost being. These moral feelings quite literally shape our experience of reality, directing our attention toward or away from what is happening around us. As one contemporary philosopher, John McMurtry, puts it, "We might best understand our human reality as a vast and complex field of values."[4] Recent research by social psychologist Jonathan Haidt[5] has helped to clarify the extent to which values are fundamental to life:

- **Values possess intuitive primacy.** People have nearly instant reactions to scenes or stories of moral violations. Affective reactions are usually good predictors of moral judgments and behaviors.
- **They guide social behavior.** When we believe that something is right, we are naturally inclined to act in a way that is consistent with this feeling.
- **They bind and build community.** Morality constrains individuals and ties them to one another to create groups. A moral community has a set of shared norms about how members ought to behave.

Where and how does this sense of intuitive primacy arise? Based on the cases that we have already cited, it is clear that the field that connects us to one another, to our family and our ancestral past, and to the wider community of all sentient life is shaped by, and sensitive to, the ethical quality of our actions as they impact others. These actions set up distinct and lasting patterns of harmony and disharmony within the field. As numerous cases from therapies such as family constellations attest, patterns of disharmony affect the health and well-being of those with a direct line of descent from whoever established the pattern in the first place. And the surfacing of these patterns also reveals the nature of, and the responsibility for, the actions that led to them. In other words, the ethical nature of the field exerts a pressure for right action and the correction of past wrongs. There is nothing new about this insight. In fact, it is one of the most ancient conceptions of ethics known to us. Some twenty-four hundred years ago, Aristotle described values as "right by nature," meaning that values are an integral part of the fabric of reality, at once absolute and universal, but at the same time variable and localized, "that which everywhere has the same force and does not exist by people's thinking this or that . . . and yet all of it is changeable."[6]

But if values are integral to and emergent from the fabric of reality, if they impart a positive force for right action and the correction of past wrongs—in short, for justice—what implications does this have for us and how we live our lives?

Integral Theory

The insight that values drive the progressive social and spiritual evolution of all sentient life occurred simultaneously to a number of thinkers around the turn of the twentieth century. In particular, Sri Aurobindo, Rudolph Steiner, Pitirim Sorokin, Jean Gebser, Ervin Laszlo, and Ken Wilber have all contributed toward developing these ideas. In the 1950s social psychologist Clare W. Graves undertook research that placed many of these ideas on a firmer basis. "Briefly, what I am proposing," he said, "is that the psychology of the mature human being is an unfolding, emergent, oscillating, spiraling process marked by progressive subordination of older, lower-order behavior systems to newer, higher-order systems as man's existential problems change."[7]

More recently, Graves's work has received confirmation from cultural anthropologist Richard Shweder.[8] A comparative analysis of moral discourse across cultures reveals that all moral discourse fits into one of three fundamental sets of values:

- the ethics of autonomy, based on such concepts as individual rights, fairness, and justice
- the ethics of community, based on duty, hierarchy, tradition, respect, and loyalty
- the ethics of divinity, based on sacred order, sanctity, and purity

Graves recognized that our moral responses manifest with a greater or lesser degree of sophistication, which represents an evolutionary factor in the unfolding of human consciousness.[9] By modulating our responses to the challenges we face in the light of our most evolved set of values, we enable healing, integration, and transformation to take place personally, societally, and globally. This evolutionary unfolding of consciousness is being played out across the entire planet. Regressive forces, such as threats to survival, whether real or imagined, can drive entire societies to enact earlier, more primitive patterns of behavior. The development of Graves's ideas into a conflict-resolution system called Spiral Dynamics[10] emphasizes the fact that only evolutionarily higher orders of ethical behavior are able to solve the increasingly complex issues facing us today.

What Can We Do?

The challenge that we all face is to realize lasting positive shifts in our psycho-energetic being. From the foregoing it should, by now, be evident that the foundation for achieving this is, first and foremost, through the integration of those emotional blockages that are holding back our progress. That said, our approach must be sufficiently nuanced to identify and counteract the consumer forces that militate against our best efforts to make progress in our personal development. We can simplify this complex process into three important categories for which we should develop definite strategies that will guide and direct our behavior:

- **Diet and exercise.** Yes, of course it is important to try to minimize our consumption of processed foods and, as much as possible, exclude them from our diet in favor of preparing organic food at home. And yes, of course an adequate amount of exercise is essential. But more significantly it is important to realize the role that junk food and beverages play in the way we manage our anxiety. Until this underlying link is tackled, other ideas about self-improvement are unlikely to lead to sustained improvement.
- **Distractions.** Ditto for digital media and other distractions. Do you find yourself spending far too much wasteful time on digital media? Again, until the link between constantly seeking distractions and their function in helping us suppress our emotions is recognized and tackled, our ideas about lasting self-improvement are unlikely to lead very far.

- **Overwork.** What we have said about distractions also goes for overworking, although admittedly there is a far more compelling rationale for overworking than for merely wasting time. Nevertheless, the same logic applies. There comes a point where work primarily serves as a way of suppressing one's feelings of anxiety.

From these three points it should be evident that our ability to identify and eliminate self-limiting patterns of behavior is a prerequisite to making progress in our personal and spiritual development. We have already mentioned the importance and usefulness of empowering oneself by mastering at least one of the now widely available energy psychology protocols. A greatly enhanced level of emotional self-management is the key to personal growth. Unless we learn to integrate our negative feelings, our goal of eliminating addictive and suppressive patterns of behavior is unlikely to be realized. The minimum adjunct to the practice of energy psychology is to learn and practice mindfulness meditation. By this I do not mean formal meditation practice—useful as that may be—but rather the habitual adoption of a state of present-moment, nonjudgmental awareness—simply breathing and observing both one's inner and outer world without spinning an internal narrative about it. This should be done routinely and at any time during the day, but especially in those situations—waiting for someone or something—that usually make us feel tense or impatient.

With these tools in hand we can start identifying those aspects of our experience that disturb us and commit to changing our relationship to them by transforming instead of acting out our reactions. The question of our relationship with those aspects of reality that we find most distasteful, or most addictive, is one of the subtlest and most complex of issues; and yet experience demonstrates that there is an intimate relationship between how we are in our innermost being and the quality of our lived experience. This relationship is such that when we change our inner reality we experience a corresponding change in our relationship with the world, and this provides us with the leverage to resculpt our lives. The question then becomes: What is the nature of the change we seek? How do we ensure that it aligns with fundamental values and supports the spiritual evolution of all sentient beings?

Eudaemonia, the Art of Human Flourishing

The starting place of ancient ethics was the search for *eudaemonia,* which means, roughly, "flourishing." In recent years positive psychology has undertaken the job of unpacking these ancient ideas and providing them with a scientific foundation. Eudaemonia is defined by Websters as "well-being," "happiness," and its benefits positively impact every single area of life without exception.[11,12]

Most of us associate or have associated happiness with external circumstances, with becoming "better off." And yet such happiness, like a mirage, always seems to recede in front of us. Studies have demonstrated that external circumstances play a very small part, around 10 to 15 percent, in our overall level of happiness. Fully half of our capacity for happiness is thought to be determined by relatively fixed factors that constitute our set point or baseline level of happiness to which we return after experiencing any high point. This only leaves around one-third of our capacity for happiness susceptible to intentional activity.[13] Clearly our set point or baseline level of happiness accounts for the majority of our reactions to life's ups and downs. Other circumstances—factors such as age, gender, education, and income—appear to have only a marginal impact. The question, therefore, is: Is it possible to increase our overall level of happiness? We need to split this question into two parts: What inner work do we need to undertake to overcome the inertia of our set point and shift our baseline level of happiness in a positive direction? And how should we manage our intentional activity to optimize eudaemonia, our happiness and flourishing?

Since consciousness exhibits a multilayered continuum (one that includes perinatal memory, past lives, and family and ancestral influences), we can use this structure to guide our inner work. Apart from our immediate senses and memory, we remain largely unconscious of the other layers. The only way we can assess the work required in each of these layers is by paying careful attention to our moment-to-moment experience. How often do we find ourselves lost in negative thoughts and feelings? What is the ratio of our negative to positive thoughts and feelings? What is the quality of our self-talk? Are there certain "tracks," narratives of self-blame and criticism that we constantly play to ourselves over and over again? Do certain recurring negative patterns keep manifesting in our relationships with loved ones or those in authority? By starting with these most mundane and yet most persistent of concerns we can begin to expand our self-awareness, and this is the prelude to enhancing our self-management. To enact self-management we should employ easy-to-use self-empowering techniques and practices such as energy psychology and mindfulness meditation. It is essential, however, that we always seek to achieve acceptance and transformation of any issue that draws our attention. For example, at the level of our present-moment awareness and biographical memory we can use the various energy psychology techniques to eliminate specific negative thoughts and feelings and replace them with positive ones; but for particularly deep issues we may need to seek an experienced professional therapist who uses energy psychology techniques. The clearing of any presenting issues can, and often does, lead to the clearing of issues at much deeper levels.

Throughout this book I have presented concrete cases of people working successfully with their underlying issues by employing a variety of approaches and techniques. Experience has shown that there are a number of golden rules that we need to bear in mind when undertaking any healing, personal development, or spiritual practices. While not exhaustive, the following principles will serve you well:

- Not all practices are suitable for us. If it doesn't feel right, listen to yourself and stop; there will be some other approach or technique that is just right for you.

- Your personal healing, self-development, or spiritual journey should not be another source of stress in your life. If it's not joyful, then it's probably the wrong thing for you.

- Not all facilitators and teachers are compatible with our personal style, no matter how highly recommended they may come. If you do not feel comfortable with someone, listen to yourself and stop; some other person will be more compatible with your personal style.

- Never try to push yourself too hard to obtain a result; everything has its own season.

- Expectations based on other people's experiences may serve as a great motivation for getting started, but we really need to keep a check on our expectations and forgo comparisons with other people. However your experience is, it's okay, that's how it was meant to be.

- Be ready to step beyond the boundaries of the known and the familiar, but recognize that each person's tolerance for the unknown and the unfamiliar is different. What is extreme for one person may be child's play for another. There is no standard against which you should measure yourself other than how you feel about it.

- Always make your best effort to transform any emotional issues that surface. Do not leave them hanging unresolved, since they will make you feel upset and unbalanced for some time afterward.

One of the reasons for emphasising the importance of remaining within one's own comfort zone when attempting any of the more energized development practices such as rebirthing breathwork or kundalini work of any kind is that the problem of retraumatization is all too often insufficiently understood or appreciated. Briefly, retraumatization occurs with any technique that causes the sudden or unexpected surfacing of a traumatic emotion from the past, but which then lacks the means to actively facilitate its integration. To the best of my knowledge, only the various energy psychology techniques can facilitate the integration of even the most traumatic of experiences. Earlier we cited clinical studies proving the success of Emotional Freedom Techniques (EFT) in providing relief to sufferers of the most extreme and intractable of anxiety disorders, post-traumatic stress disorder (PTSD), as proof of this. If you can achieve a higher degree of emotional self-management through energy psychology, then you will be better equipped to handle anything that arises during the course of your inner work.

Apart from our personal development work we need to look at the texture of our day-to-day lives. Positive psychology provides a useful framework that we can readily adopt. Its research suggests that human flourishing arises from the managed convergence of three related life strategies: the pleasant life, or life of enjoyment; the good life, or life of engagement; and the meaningful life, or life of affiliation.[14]

The pleasant life consists of simply having as many pleasurable experiences as possible. Few of us would object to this idea. However, as a life strategy this approach alone doesn't lead to a stable sense of personal fulfillment or enduring happiness. It has been found that after some months, even lottery winners revert to much the same (and sometimes an even worse) emotional state than before they won the lottery.[15] From an early age, most of us are, to some degree, addicted to the pleasant life. It is, after all, the force that drives consumerism. But its satisfactions are, inevitably, transitory. The evaporation of the emotional high associated with new experiences leaves us once more face-to-face with ourselves, our raw state of being or set point to which we return again and again. When pursued to the exclusion of all else, the pleasant life is also the dissatisfied life. Boredom drives an endless search for new sources of stimulation. Fortunately, this is not the only strategy open to us. If we enjoy our pleasures and yet remain unfulfilled, then we need to look to the next level—to the good life.

The good life involves deep engagement with our work and our family life, or indeed any other activities that give rise to a profound sense of personal satisfaction and fulfillment. All of the available research agrees that our relationships with our family and friends are one of the most important contributors to our overall level of happiness. Parallel to these are all of the other areas of life with which we are involved. In particular, our work life absorbs most of our waking hours. To engage deeply with something we need to be able to apply our most defining strengths and capabilities, sometimes known as "signature strengths,"[16] to it. Using our core strengths and capabilities gives rise to a sense of well-being that is anchored in the deepest levels of our being. Applying yourself completely to something that fully engages your strengths typically leads to a state of complete absorption called *flow*.[17] Flow is a state that people experience when they are completely absorbed in what they are doing to the point of forgetting time, fatigue, and everything else but what they are doing. The experience of flow has been described as:

> being completely involved in an activity for its own sake. The ego falls away. Time flies. Every action, movement, and thought follows inevitably from the previous one, like playing jazz. Your whole being is involved, and you're using your skills to the utmost.[18]

If you have never experienced flow or only infrequently experience it, then you probably need to check what your signature strengths are.[19, 20] Look at how you are using them on a day-to-day basis and begin to resculpt your life to engage more of your strengths more fully more of the time. But even attaining the "good" or engaged life may still not provide the sense of purpose and fulfillment that we seek. "Just as well-being needs to be anchored in strengths and virtues, these in turn must be anchored in something larger. Just as the good life is something beyond the pleasant life, the meaningful life is beyond the good life."[21]

The meaningful life consists in placing our signature strengths in the service of a cause larger than ourselves. We derive a positive sense of well-being, belonging, meaning, and purpose from being part of and contributing to something larger and more permanent (e.g., nature, charity and community groups, organizations, movements, and belief systems). One area in which these higher levels of engagement emerge is in authentic leadership. Major life challenges have the potential to generate an inner transformation characterized as moving from an "I" to a "we" perspective,[22] a shift in orientation from service to self, to service to others. Moving from focusing on one's own private goals and targets to taking responsibility for the collective and for serving its goals and objectives, even at personal cost, has been called "entering the fundamental state of leadership."[23] It is characterized as:

- moving beyond one's comfort zone to explore new possibilities
- acting from one's core values rather than conforming to other's expectations
- acting for the collective good rather than pursuing self-interest
- embracing change rather than relying on routines

On this planet we are faced with enormous challenges, but through these we can see, if only dimly, the outlines of a future humanity existing on a higher arc of spiritual evolution. The task of realizing this future is not someone else's. It is certainly not the task of some remote political or corporate elite. The task of realizing this better future is yours and mine and all of us who wish for something better, not only for ourselves and our loved ones, but for all sentient life. By opening ourselves to the power of love and by taking responsibility for our own healing, all contribute directly to the harmony of the larger field. After all, we are, all of us, a part of a much greater whole.

Notes

Chapter 1. Healing, Energy, and Consciousness

1. Nagel, *Mind and Cosmos,* 61–65, 86–87.
2. Kauffman, *Reinventing the Sacred,* 6–9.
3. Ludwig, "Altered states."
4. Tart, *Altered States,* 2.
5. Krippner, "Altered States," 1, 5.
6. Ehrmann, "Some critical issues."

Chapter 2. Psi and Intuitive Knowledge

1. Haraldsson et al., "Psychic experience."
2. Levin, "Age differences."
3. Sheldrake, "Dog that seems to know."
4. Breen, "Nature, Incidence."
5. Miller, *Dowsing,* 20.
6. Betz, "Unconventional water detection."
7. Laughlin, "Consciousness."
8. Taylor, *Secular Age,* 329.
9. Lumpkin, "Perceptual Diversity and Its Implications."
10. Lumpkin, "Is polyphasic consciousness necessary."
11. Plato, *Theaetetus,* 201c–d.
12. Ayer, *Problem of Knowledge,* 128–161.
13. Katz, *Boiling Energy.*
14. Lewis-Williams, *Mind,* 193–196.

15. Hadot, *Philosophy*, 81–125.
16. Foucault, *Hermeneutics*, 17.

Chapter 3. Healing Issues within Our Timeline

1. Grof, *Holotropic Mind*, 34.
2. Turner and Turner, "Rebirthing."
3. Chopra, *The Essential*, 103.
4. Seto et al., "Detection."
5. Kokubo, "Concept of 'Qi.'"
6. Ma, "Roots."
7. Dorfer et al., "Medical report," 1023–1026.
8. Dorfer et al., "Medical report," 1023.
9. Church et al., "Psychological symptom change."
10. Church, "Treatment of combat trauma."
11. Church et al., "Psychological trauma symptom improvement."
12. Davidson et al., "Alterations."
13. Davidson and Lutz, "Buddha's brain."
14. Fredrickson, "Broaden-and-build."

Chapter 4. Healing Issues beyond Our Timeline

1. Hellinger, *Love's Hidden Symmetry*.

Chapter 5. The Healing Field

1. Nagel, *Mind and Cosmos*, 66–67, 91–93.
2. Grof, *Holotropic Mind*, 33–79.
3. Stevenson, "Birthmarks."
4. Pasricha, "Some bodily malformations."
5. Hellinger, *Love's Hidden Symmetry*.
6. Clark and Chalmers, "The extended mind."
7. Quoted in International Systemic Constellations Association, "Systemic Constellations."
8. Sheldrake, *Morphic Resonance*.
9. Sheldrake, "Morphic Resonance and Morphic Fields."

10. Sheldrake, "Morphic Resonance and Morphic Fields."
11. Dawkins, *Selfish Gene,* 192.
12. Beck and Cowan, *Spiral Dynamics,* 31–33.
13. Sheldrake, *Presence,* 223–238.
14. Plato, *Phaedrus,* 244d.
15. Rich and Merchant, "Rupert Sheldrake."
16. Stavish, *Egregores.*
17. Aardema, *Explorations,* 201–232.
18. Sinclair, *Sword and the Grail,* 165.

Chapter 6. Healing on Extended Planes of Existence

1. Turner, *Experiencing Ritual,* 149.
2. Turner, *Experiencing Ritual,* 149.
3. Turner, "The reality of spirits," 9.
4. Grindal, "Into the heart," 68.
5. Grindal, "Into the heart," 76.
6. Sogyal Rinpoche, *Tibetan Book of Living and Dying.*
7. Maté, *In the Realm of Hungry Ghosts,* 197–201.
8. Sagan, *Entity Possession.*
9. Greenwood, "Possession."
10. Fiore, *Unquiet Dead.*
11. Sanderson, "Case for Spirit Release."
12. Modi, *Remarkable Healings.*
13. Baldwin and Fiore, *Spirit Releasement.*
14. Greenwood, "Possession."
15. Vallée and Davis, "Incommensurability."

Chapter 7. Healing through Spirit

1. Tierney, "Hallucinogens."
2. Maslow, *Religions.*
3. Pew Research Center, "Second annual poll."
4. James, *Varieties,* 257–292.
5. Happold, *Mysticism.*
6. Shrader, "Seven Characteristics."

7. Underhill, *Mysticism,* 165–166.

8. John of the Cross, *Dark Night.*

9. Merton, *New Man,* 19.

10. Wong, *Cultivating,* 54.

11. Forman, "What does mysticism have to teach."

12. Lao Tse, *Tao Te Ching.*

13. Vaughan, *Henry Vaughan,* 113.

14. Quoted in Schultes et al., *Plants of the Gods,* 3.

15. Fermor, *Time to Keep Silence,* 1.

16. Katz, *Boiling Energy,* 94.

17. Katz, "Painful Ecstasy," 168.

18. Sopa, "Subtle Body," 144.

19. Grof, "Frontiers."

20. Johnson, "Reflections."

21. Zimmerman, "Laying-on-of-hands."

22. Seto et al., "Detection."

23. Herron-Marx et al., "Systematic review."

24. Norbu, *Crystal,* 33.

25. Cicero, *On the Commonwealth,* 143–144.

26. Kerenyi, *Eleusis,* 12.

27. Van Gennep, *Rites of Passage,* 21.

28. Burkert, *Ancient Mystery Cults,* 90–91.

Chapter 8. Conclusions

1. Forman, *An Emerging New Model,* 279–299.

2. Goswami, *The Physicists',* 279–288.

3. MacIntyre, *After Virtue,* 3.

4. McMurtry, "Philosophy," 8.

5. Haidt, "New synthesis."

6. Aristotle, *Complete Works,* 1790–1.

7. Graves, "Human Nature."

8. Shweder et al., "'Big Three.'"

9. Graves, "Human Nature."

10. Beck and Cowan, *Spiral Dynamics.*

11. Fredrickson, "Broaden-and-build."

12. Fredrickson and Losada, "Positive affect."

13. Lyubomirsky et al., "Pursuing happiness."

14. Seligman, *Authentic Happiness,* 13–14.

15. Brickman et al., "Lottery winners."

16. Seligman and Peterson, *Character Strengths,* 13–14.

17. Csikszentmihalyi, *Flow.*

18. Geirland, "Go."

19. Niemiec and McGrath, *The Power of Character Strengths.*

20. VIA Signature Strengths Survey at: www.authentichappiness.com.

21. Seligman, *Authentic Happiness,* 14.

22. George, *Discover Your True North,* 181–198.

23. Quinn, "Moments," 74.

Bibliography

Aardema, Fredrick. *Explorations in Consciousness: A New Approach to Out-of-Body Experiences*. Quebec, Canada: Mount Royal Publishing, 2012.

Aristotle. *The Complete Works of Aristotle, Volume 2*. Ed. Jonathan Barnes. Princeton: N.J., 1984.

Ayer, Alfred. *The Problem of Knowledge*. London: Macmillan & Co. Ltd., New York: St. Martin's Press, 1956.

Baldwin, William and Edith Fiore. *Spirit Releasement Therapy: A Technique Manual*. London: Headline Press, 1995.

Beck, Don Edward and Christopher C. Cowan. *Spiral Dynamics: Mastering Values, Leadership, and Change*. Hoboken: Wiley-Blackwell, 1996.

Betz, Hans-Dieter. "Unconventional water detection: Field test of the dowsing technique in dry zones." *Journal of Scientific Exploration* 9, no. 1 (1995): 1–43.

Breen, Rosemary. "The Nature, Incidence, and Impact of Paranormal Experiences: An Exploratory Mixed Methods Research Study." Monash University thesis, 2019.

Brickman, Philip, Dan Coates, and Ronnie Janoff-Bulman. "Lottery winners and accident victims: Is happiness relative?" *Journal of Personality and Social Psychology* 36, no. 8 (1978): 917–27.

Burkert, Walter. *Ancient Mystery Cults*. Cambridge, Mass.: Harvard University Press, 1987.

Chopra, Deepak. *The Essential Ageless Body, Timeless Mind: The Essence of the Quantum Alternative to Growing Old*. New York: Harmony, 2007.

Church, Dawson. "Treatment of combat trauma in veterans using EFT: A pilot protocol." *Traumatology* 16, no.1 (2010): 55–65.

———, Linda Geronilla, and Ingrid Dinter. "Psychological symptom change in veterans after six sessions of Emotional Freedom Techniques (EFT): An observational study." *International Journal of Healing and Caring* 9, no. 1 (2009).

———, Crystal Hawk, Audrey J. Brooks, Olli Toukolehto, Mario Wren, Ingrid Dinter, and Phyllis Stein. "Psychological trauma symptom improvement in veterans using Emotional Freedom Techniques: A randomized controlled trial." *Journal of Nervous and Mental Disease* 201, no. 2 (2013): 153–60.

Cicero, Marcus Tullius. *Cicero: On the Commonwealth and On the Laws (Cambridge Texts in the History of Political Thought)*. Trans. James E. G. Zetzel. Cambridge: Cambridge University Press, 2017.

Clark, Andy and David Chalmers. "The extended mind." *Analysis* 58, no. 1 (1998): 10–23.

Csikszentmihalyi, Mikhail. *Flow: The Psychology of Optimal Experience.* New York: Harper Perennial Modern Classics, 2008.

Davidson, Richard, Jon Kabat-Zinn, Jessica Schumacher, Melissa Rosenkranz, Daniel Muller, Saki F. Santorelli, Ferris Urbanowski, Anne Harrington, Katherine Bonus, and John F. Sheridan. "Alterations in brain and immune function produced by mindfulness meditation." *Psychosomatic Medicine* 65, no. 4 (2003): 564–70.

Davidson, Richard and Antoine Lutz. "Buddha's brain: Neuroplasticity and meditation." *IEEE Signal Processing Magazine* 25, no. 1 (2008): 174–76.

Dawkins, Richard. *The Selfish Gene.* Oxford, U.K.: Oxford University Press, 1976.

Dorfer, L., M. Moser, F. Bahr, K. Spindler, E. Egarter-Vigl, S. Giullen, G. Dohr, and T. Kenner. "A medical report from the stone age?" *Lancet* 354, no. 9183 (1999): 1023–25.

Ehrmann, Wilfried. "Some critical issues in Stan and Christina Grof's holotropic breathwork: A discussion between Wilfried Ehrmann and Stan Grof M.D." *Healing Breath* 3, no. 3, (2001).

Fermor, Patrick. *A Time to Keep Silence.* London: John Murray, 2004.

Fiore, Edith. *The Unquiet Dead: A Psychologist Treats Spirit Possession.* New York: Doubleday, 1987.

Forman, Robert K. C. "An Emerging New Model for Consciousness: The Consciousness Field Model." In *Neuroscience, Consciousness and*

Spirituality. Ed. H. Walach, S. Schmidt, W. B. Jonas. Dordrecht: Springer Netherlands, 2008.

———. "What does mysticism have to teach us about consciousness?" *Journal of Consciousness Studies* 5, no. 2 (1998): 185–201.

Foucault, Michel. *The Hermeneutics of the Subject: Lectures at the College de France 1981–82*. London: Picador, 2005.

Fredrickson, Barbara. "The broaden-and-build theory of positive emotions." *Philosophical Transactions of the Royal Society of London Series B: Biological Sciences* 359, no. 1449 (2004): 1367–77.

——— and Marsial Losada. "Positive affect and the complex dynamics of human flourishing." *American Psychologist* 60, no. 7 (2005): 678–86.

Geirland, John. "Go with the Flow." *Wired*, September 1, 1996.

George, William. *Discover Your True North*. Hoboken: Jossey-Bass, 2015.

Goswami, Amit. *The Physicists' View of Nature Part 2: The Quantum Revolution*. Berlin: Springer, 2002.

Graves, Clare. "Human nature prepares for a momentous leap." *Futurist*, April (1974): 72–87.

Greenwood, Michael. "Possession." *Medical Acupuncture* 20, no. 1 (2008): 23–32.

Grindal, Bruce. "Into the heart of Sisala experience: Witnessing death divination." *Journal of Anthropological Research* 39, no. 1 (1983): 60–80.

Grof, Stanislav. "Frontiers of the mind: Interview with Stanislav Grof MD." Interview by Daniel Redwood (2013), Awaken.com.

Grof, Stanislav. *The Holotropic Mind: The Three Levels of Human Consciousness and How They Shape Our Lives*. San Francisco, Calif.: HarperOne, 1992.

Hadot, Pierre. *Philosophy as a Way of Life: Spiritual Exercises from Socrates to Foucault*. Malden, Mass.: Blackwell, 1995.

Haidt, Jon. "The new synthesis in moral psychology." *Science* 316, no. 5827 (2007): 998–1002.

Happold, Frederick. *Mysticism*. London: Penguin Books, 1991.

Haraldsson, Erlendur and Joop M. Hootkouper. "Psychic experience in the multinational human values study: Who reports them?" *Journal of the American Society for Psychical Research* 85, no. 2 (1991): 145–65.

Hellinger, Bert, Gunthard Weber, and Hunter Beaumont. *Love's Hidden Symmetry: What Makes Love Work in Relationships*. Phoenix, Ariz.: Zeig, Tucker & Theisen Inc., 1998.

Herron-Marx, Sandy, Femke Knol, Barbara Burden, and Carolyn Hicks. "A systematic review of the use of Reiki in health care." *Alternative and Complementary Therapies* 14, no. 1 (2008): 37–42.

International Systemic Constellations Association. "Systemic Constellations." ISCA-Network.org.

James, William. *The Varieties of Religious Experience*. London: Penguin Classics, 1985.

John of the Cross. *Dark Night of the Soul,* New York: Dover Publications, 2003.

Johnson, Chad. "Reflections on a silent meditation retreat: A beginner's perspective." *International Journal of Transpersonal Studies* 28 (2009): 134–38.

Katz, Richard. *Boiling Energy: Community Healing among the Kalahari Kung*. Cambridge, Mass.: Harvard University Press, 1982.

———. "The Painful Ecstasy of Healing," 165–169 in Daniel Goleman and Richard Davidson, eds., *Consciousness: Brain, States of Awareness and Mysticism*. New York: Harper & Row, 1979.

Kauffman, Stuart. *Reinventing the Sacred: A New View of Science, Reason, and Religion*. New York: Basic Books, 2008.

Kerenyi, Carl. *Eleusis: Archetypal Image of Mother and Daughter*. Princeton, N.J.: Princeton Univerity Press, 1991.

Kokubo, Hideyuki. "Concept of 'Qi' or 'Ki' in Japanese Qigong Research." Proceedings of the 44th Annual Convention of the Parapsychological Association. New York, 2001: 147–54.

Krippner, Stanley. "Altered States of Consciousness," in John White, ed., *The Highest State of Consciousness*. Guildford, U.K.: White Crow Books, 2012.

Lao Tse. *Tao Te Ching*. New York: Harper Perennial, 2006.

Laughlin, Charles. "Consciousness in biogenetic structural theory." *Anthropology of Consciousness* 3, no. 1–2 (1992): 17–22.

Levin, Jeffrey. "Age differences in mystical experience." *Gerontologist* 33, no. 4 (1993): 507–13.

Lewis-Williams, David. *The Mind in the Cave: Consciousness and the Origins of Art*. London: Thames & Hudson, 2002.

Ludwig, Arnold. "Altered states of consciousness." *Archives of General Psychiatry* 15, no. 3 (1966): 225–34.

Lumpkin, Tara Waters. "Perceptual Diversity and Its Implications for Development: A Case Study of Namibian Traditional Medicine." Ph.D. dissertation, Union Institute, March 31, 1996.

————. "Perceptual diversity: Is polyphasic consciousness necessary for global survival?" *Anthropology of Consciousness* 12, no. 1 (2001): 37–70.

Lyubomirsky, Sonja, Kennon M. Sheldon, and David Schkade. "Pursuing happiness: The architecture of sustainable change." *Review of General Psychology* 9, no. 2 (2005): 111–31.

MacIntyre, Alistair. *After Virtue: A Study in Moral Theory.* Notre Dame, Ind.: University of Notre Dame Press, 2007.

Ma, Kan-Wen. "The roots and development of Chinese acupuncture: From prehistory to early 20th century." *Acupuncture in Medicine* 10, 1 suppl. (1992): 92–99.

Maslow, Abraham. *Religions, Values and Peak Experiences.* New York: Penguin, 1994.

Maté, Gabor. *In the Realm of Hungry Ghosts: Close Encounters with Addiction.* Berkeley, Calif.: North Atlantic Books, 2010.

McMurtry, John, *Philosophy and World Problems Vol. 1 The Global Crisis of Values.* UNESCO-EOLSS, 2002.

Merton, Thomas. *The New Man.* New York: Farrar, Straus and Giroux, 1999.

Miller, Hamish. *Dowsing: A Journey Beyond Our Five Senses.* Bury St. Edmunds: Wooden Books, 2007.

Modi, Shakuntala. *Remarkable Healings: A Psychiatrist Discovers Unsuspected Roots of Mental and Physical Illness.* Charlottesville, Va.: Hampton Roads Publishing Co., Inc., 1997.

Nagel, Thomas. *Mind and Cosmos: Why the Materialist Neo-Darwinian Conception of Nature Is Almost Certainly False.* New York: Oxford University Press, 2012.

Niemiec, Ryan M. and Robert E. McGrath. *The Power of Character Strengths: Appreciate and Ignite Your Positive Personality.* Cincinnati, Ohio: VIA Institute on Character, 2019.

Norbu, Chögyal Namkhai. *The Crystal and the Way of Light: Sutra, Tantra and Dzogchen.* Ithaca, N.Y.: Snow Lion, 1986, 2000.

Pasricha, Satwant, Jurgen Keil, Jim Tucker, and Ian Stevenson. "Some bodily malformations attributed to previous lives." *Journal of Scientific Exploration* 19, no. 3 (2005): 359–83.

Pew Research Center. "Pew Forum and Pew Research Center release second annual poll." (2002) PewForum.org.

Plato. *Phaedrus.* Trans. Paul Woodruff and Alexander Nehamas. Cambridge, MA: Hackett Publishing Co., 1995.

———. *Theaetetus.* Available at Perseus.tufts.edu.

Quinn, Robert. "Moments of greatness: Entering the fundamental state of leadership." *Harvard Business Review* 83, no. 7 (2005): 74–83.

Rich, Paul and David Merchant. "Rupert Sheldrake and the search for morphic resonances." *Contemporary Philosophy* 22 (2000): 453–44.

Sagan, Samuel. *Entity Possession: Freeing the Energy Body of Negative Influences.* Rochester, Vt.: Destiny Books, 1997.

Sanderson, Alan. "The Case for Spirit Release." *Royal College of Psychiatry, Spirituality Special Interest Group* (SSIG), 2003.

Schultes, Richard, Albert Hofmann, and Christian Rätsch. *Plants of the Gods: Their Sacred, Healing, and Hallucinogenic Powers.* Rochester, Vt.: Healing Arts Press, 2001.

Seligman, Martin. *Authentic Happiness: Using the New Positive Psychology to Realize Your Potential for Lasting Fulfillment.* New York: Atria Books, 2005.

——— and Christopher Peterson. *Character Strengths and Virtues: A Handbook and Classification.* Washington D.C., American Psychological Association: Oxford University Press, 2004.

Seto, Akira, C. Kusaka, S. Nakazato, W. R. Huang, T. Sato, T. Hisamitsu, and C. Takeshige. "Detection of extraordinary large bio-magnetic field strength from human hand during external Qi emission." *Acupuncture and Electrotherapeutics Research* 17, no. 2 (1992): 72–94.

Sheldrake, Rupert. "A dog that seems to know when his owner is coming home: Videotaped experiments and observations." *Journal of Scientific Exploration* 14, no. 2 (2000): 233–55.

———. *Morphic Resonance: The Nature of Formative Causation.* Rochester, Vt.: Park Street Press, 2009.

———. "Morphic Resonance and Morphic Fields." At www.sheldrake.org.

———. *The Presence of the Past: Morphic Resonance and the Habits of Nature.* Rochester, Vt.: Park Street Press, 2012.

Shrader, Douglas. "The Seven Characteristics of Mystical Experience." Proceedings of the 6th Annual Hawaii International Conference on Arts and Humanities. Honolulu, Hawaii, 2008.

Shweder, Richard A., Nancy C. Much, Manamohan Mahapatra, and Lawrence Park. "The 'Big Three' of Morality (Autonomy, Community, Divinity) and the 'Big Three' Explanations of Suffering," 119–69, in Allan M. Brandt and Paul Rozin, eds., *Morality and Health*. New York and London: Routledge, 1997.

Sinclair, Andrew. *The Sword and the Grail: The Story of the Grail, the Templars and the True Discovery of America*. Edinburgh, Scotland: Birlinn Publishing, 2002.

Sogyal Rinpoche. *The Tibetan Book of Living and Dying*. San Francisco: HarperOne, 1992.

Sopa, Geshe Lhundub. "The Subtle Body in Tantric Buddhism," 139–158, in Geshe Lhundub Sopa, Roger Jackson, and John Newman, eds., *The Wheel of Time: The Kalachakra in Context*. Ithaca, N.Y.: Snow Lion, 1985, 1991.

Stavish, Mark. *Egregores: The Occult Entities That Watch Over Human Destiny*. Rochester, Vt.: Inner Traditions, 2018.

Stevenson, Ian. "Birthmarks and birth defects corresponding to wounds on deceased persons." *Journal of Scientific Exploration* 7, no. 4 (1993): 403–10.

Tart, Charles, ed. *Altered States of Consciousness: A Book of Readings*. New York: Doubleday, 1972.

Taylor, Charles. *A Secular Age*. Cambridge, Mass.: Belknap Press of Harvard University Press, 2018.

Tierney, John. "Hallucinogens Have Doctors Tuning In Again." *New York Times,* April 11, 2010.

Tressoldi, P. E., M. Martinelli, S. Massaccesi, and L. Sartori. "Heart rate differences between targets and non-targets in intuitive tasks." *Human Physiology* 31, no. 6 (2005): 646–50.

Turner, Edith. "The reality of spirits." *Shamanism* 10, no.1 (1997).

———, with William Blodgett, Singleton Kahona, and Fideli Benwa. *Experiencing Ritual: A New Interpretation of African Healing*. Philadelphia, Pa.: University of Pennsylvania Press, 1992.

Turner, Jon and Troya Turner. "Rebirthing or rebreathing: A recapitulation." *Healing Breath* 2, no. 3 (2000): 22–37.